C-Section Recovery Manual

Your Body
Your Recovery

Janine McKnight Cowan and Leonie Rastas

C-Section Recovery Manual: Your Body, Your Recovery
© Leonie Rastas and Janine McKnight-Cowan 2022

ISBN: 978-1-922461-95-7 (Paperback)
         978-1-922461-98-8 (eBook)

A catalogue record for this book is available from the National Library of Australia

Editors: Kristy Martin and Jason Martin
Proofread by: Sarah Kate Hill
Cover Design: Emily Rastas and Ocean Reeve Publishing
Photography: Jessica Vink Netherlands
Design and Typeset: Ocean Reeve Publishing
Printed in Australia by Ocean Reeve Publishing

Published by Leonie Rastas, Janine McKnight-Cowan, and Ocean Reeve Publishing
www.oceanreevepublishing.com

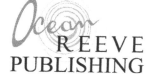

This manual belongs to: _____

It was purchased by: _____

My C-section date: _____

My baby's/babies' name/s:_____

Born on:_____ Time: _____ Weight: _____

My pregnancy was_____ weeks long.

I had a C-section due to: _____

'What matters to me in my postpartum recovery is ...'

Examples:

- I eat well, I ask for help, I ask those caring for me to ask me 'what matters to me'.

- I have a postnatal plan to document my wishes and names of my support team.

- I want to understand what normal healing looks like and I know when to consult the doctor.

- My baby is not kissed or handled by visitors.

- I want to resist the temptation to 'bounce back' and rather give myself permission to have a slow postpartum, so I can spend quality time bonding with my baby and allowing my body to heal.

Other:

_____

_____

_____

Reviews

The purpose of this manual is to help equip you to understand the why, when, how, *and* what *happens to you and your body during and following Caesarean section surgery.*

Janine and Leonie have aimed to cover all the trade learnt personal and professional experiences that they have seen over eighty-five years of practice collectively. Furthermore, they help you to understand the anatomy and physiology of your caesarean birth, and why specific care is recommended.

Creative and practical daily planners will aid the preparation for your recovery from Caesarean section to ensure it is a smooth, safe and productive life experience.

The journals you will have always to reflect on, this is essential to record minute by minute, hour by hour and day by day positive reinforcement of your time as a new parent.

—Jeanna Partridge, A UK-based Registered General Nurse twenty-one-year practising midwife with qualifications, (BSc (Hons) Midwifery), post-graduate diploma, and experience as a specialist community public health nurse/health visitor.

I wish I had C-Section Recovery Manual: Your Body, Your Recovery *after I experienced my first birth: a slightly traumatic emergency C-section. I was completely unprepared for the recovery journey in the days, weeks and months, post birth. I underestimated the impact of the birth and wasn't equipped with how to care and support my body.*

Now that I've been through three C-sections, I know the recovery can look different with each birth, and the difference between a planned C-Section and an emergency one is vastly different. Having a resource like C-section Recovery Manual: Your Body, Your Recovery *would definitely help mums with their post C-Section journey.*

C-Section Recovery Manual Your Body, Your Recovery is comprehensive, easy to read, and answers every question you might have about the surgery and post-birth experience. It's full of useful information and tools to help navigate what can be an overwhelming time.

It's well-researched and draws on the author's vast knowledge on the subject.

I would recommend it to anyone who is planning a C-Section, or any Mum who finds herself birthing via emergency C-Section.

—Alison Meredith, three-time C-Section mother

Thank you to Leonie and Janine. Finally, there is a concise resource for women having a caesarean birth. The C-Section Recovery Manual is a very informative, highly sensitive, and enlightening book.

I was diagnosed with a placenta praevia at 23 weeks and hospitalised for 3 months to await a caesarean birth. The void of information to help prepare for, or recover from, the surgery was alarming. Looking back the C-section was a lonely space and disempowering in many ways. It should not have been like this. I am delighted that women can now journey with Leonie and Janine's recovery manual.

Recovery from a caesarean is a mind, body, and soul experience. Being surrounded by the right people and having quality information can save unnecessary stress.
Managing post-surgery pain, negotiating breastfeeding managing the baby's needs, coping with emotions, handling family responsibilities and meeting community expectations can be overwhelming.

Apart from the clear information and gentle guidance in the C- Section manual there are wonderful tips and ideas about best standard preparation and recovery.

Whether it's your first or subsequent caesarean birth, having this manual to accompany you is like having a good friend

—**Glenda Anderson,** C-section mother

C-Section Recovery Manual: Your Body, Your Recovery *is a comprehensive and informative guide for any mother who is considering or who has experienced a C-section. Leonie and Janine have thought of every aspect of the journey, from pain and scar management, right through to what to expect when breastfeeding. Their passion for new mothers from a biopsychosocial perspective is evident throughout the manual.*

The journals and daily planners are empowering tools that provide valuable information for first time mothers and as a point of reference and reflection after a second, third, or even fourth birth!

As a health professional, I love the fact that Your Body, Your Recovery *delivers all of the information you could possibly want, in addition to facts and tips that you may not have even considered prior to birthing a baby via C-section. This is a must-read for anyone looking for an evidence-based and pragmatic guide to C-sections.*

—**Sophie Garrity** BAppSc(HM) Doctor of Physiotherapy

My three babies were all Caesarean births. The C-section recovery manual helped me better understand the process I went through and to validate some of my feelings at the time. I learnt a lot of things that I hadn't known about my surgeries like the layers that are cut through and explanations for the advice to take it easy for six weeks. It was interesting to see the list of advantages and disadvantages for caesarean birth for the first time. At times I felt tearful realising the important things both myself and family were unaware of in relation to my recovery and healing. I found the stories and examples from the author's collective midwifery experiences were helpful in explaining the needs of women after caesarean birth.

Leonie and Janine's book is an important manual not only for the mother but her partner, family, and friends to help them understand how they can be the best support during the recovery period. The book gives deep insight into the whole surgical process and healing phase. I'd highly recommend this book for any C-section mum, her partner and anyone else in her support network. Actually, I think every woman who has to have a C-section should have a C-section recovery manual on her bedside table!

—**Lizzie Child**, three-time C-section mother

Disclaimer

The content of this manual contains opinions and educational knowledge for the purpose of caesarean section recovery. This manual is not intended to provide specific diagnosis, treatment, or medical assessment. Any products or recommendations of services are for information and educational purposes only. The information within cannot be specific to your individual circumstance; you should only rely on this information to support you in making an informed decision that does not replace professional medical advice diagnosis or treatment. This manual creates a virtual patient-healthcare provider relationship, based upon the authors' dual narratives drawn from clinical practice and professional education acquired jointly over eighty-five years of midwifery maternal practice.

Developments in medical research and/or technology may impact the health or medical information provided herein. No assurance can be given that the information contained in this manual will always include the most recent findings or developments with respect to the material. Do not disregard, avoid, or delay obtaining medical or health-related advice from your healthcare professional purely on the content provided in this manual.

Please consult your general practitioner or healthcare provider regarding any medical or health-related diagnosis, treatment options, or procedures. If you believe you or any other individual has a medical emergency or any other health problem, you should promptly call an emergency medical service provider or consult a healthcare professional. The authors have developed this manual to support you to make an informed choice about your wellbeing.

About the authors

Leonie Rastas Fellow ACN, Cert Midwifery, Cert General Nursing, GradCert HE, Cert Clinical Pastoral Education. Cert IV Training & Assessment

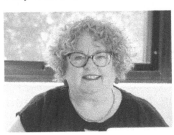 Leonie birthed her own six children all via caesarean section and she is passionate about helping support women with their recovery after a surgical birth. She is motivated by her core values of compassion, justice, respect, and dignity for all. Her quest is to help bridge the acknowledged gap in post-caesarean-birth support. Her hope is that mothers will feel, proud, and confident as they begin the healing process and bonding and attachment with their baby.

Leonie has worked as a nurse and midwife since 1977 and was admitted as a Fellow of the Australian College of Nursing in 2010 for her service to holistic healthcare. She also holds a Graduate Certificate in Higher Education, teaching nurses and midwives at tertiary level for ten years and speaking internationally.

Leonie designed a wound splint in 2018—the surgical aftercare (SAC) splint, which has been approved by the Australian Therapeutic Goods Administration for use as a medical aid and was shortlisted in Australian Healthcare Innovation awards in 2019.

Over the years, Leonie has established two healthcare organisations. Pastoral Healthcare Network Australia in 2005, a health promotion charity offering holistic healthcare for people living with grief loss and social isolation. <Caesarcare.com> was established in 2018 as a childbirth education resource and support service for women recovering from a surgical birth. Leonie believes this to be important for all mothers but be especially for any who may be feeling overwhelmed after emergency C-section births.

Leonie ponders how different mother-baby bonding and attachment could be if all C-section mammas had access to better resources to support and guide them through their postpartum.

She is passionate about helping women who birth via C-section to experience equity in childbirth education and has joined with co-author and kindred spirit Janine McKnight-Cowan to write the *C-section Recovery Manual: Your Body, Your Recovery*.

Janine McKnight-Cowan BEM, BSc Hons Midwifery, BSc Hons SCPHN, RGN, Dip HE Critical Care, Queens Nurse

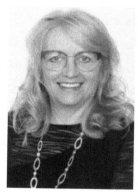

Janine also holds a Bachelor of Science with Honours in Midwifery from Birmingham University and a Bachelor of Science with Honours in Public Health Nursing from Wolverhampton University.

Janine first qualified as a registered general nurse back in 1980, going on to celebrate forty-two years of National Health Service career in the United Kingdom. Her practices have been in general nursing, midwifery, and community public health.

She has won accolades in the United Kingdom, including *Nursing Times* Team Award 2006, Queen's Nurse award for Community Nursing in 2010, Royal College of Nursing Celebrating Nursing Practice Award 2017, Royal College of Nursing Innovation and Royal College of Nursing Foundation Award 2018, and Royal College of Nursing Community & General Practice Nurse of the Year Award 2019. In 2019, Her Majesty Queen Elizabeth conferred to Janine the British Empire Medal (Civil Division) for Services to Nursing.

She is currently still practicing as a Personalised Care project manager within the NHS. Working constantly as an advocate for maternity community health as a speaker, educator, and now published author.

She is the author and innovator of the 'Five Guide' C-section recovery tool, used within this manual.

Mother to grown-up sons, and a grandmother, she describes herself as 'The clinician and woman I would want to take home with me following childbirth, so I can continue to be cared for well and recover to my best ability whilst navigating the new role of motherhood.'

Contents

Acknowledgements

This project has been a labour of love for us. We have both worked with women preparing for C-section for many years and have identified a need for targeted education and support for surgical birth. We met at the International Maternity Expo in November 2019 in London and formed a strong connection even though we had only just met. We bonded over our passion for enhancing caesarean care.

Our C-section recovery manual is our expression of our love and care for women. It is also our legacy from our midwifery careers.

Janine

For me, the greatest joy in my whole career was as a midwife—I was truly a mother's advocate. Supporting her through her labour and delivery changed me as a woman, as a mother, and as a daughter, respecting more my own mother, who delivered all five of her babies at home. For the babies I delivered and the women I cared for, safety, compassion, and respect has always been my focus. No matter how tired I ever was, whatever time of day or night it was, my focus was on a safe outcome for all.

This book is a legacy and is written with you all in mind. Now, as my own grandchildren are born—some by C-section—it is for them and all mothers who have surgical births.

Leonie

I will be forever thankful to my children—Michael, David, Karin, Nick, Tom, and Emily—all born by C-section, and who helped me to learn so much more than I'd learnt in the textbooks. For my amazing husband, Veijo, who supported me through six caesarean recoveries, always believed in me, and kept the home fires burning during the writing process for this manual. My first C-section was performed at forty-one weeks gestation, after an induction or labour was cancelled owing to my baby's head being high and mobile. An X-ray of my pelvic bones was then ordered, identifying cephalopelvic disproportion (CPD), meaning baby's head could not fit through the pelvis.

My next five babies were born by repeat caesarean section as it was pretty much the norm for the time. 'Once a caesarean, always a caesarean.' My birthing journey over fifteen years presented many challenges and complications, all of which have positively influenced my empathy and passionate desire to help women preparing for and recovering from a surgical birth.

Personally, I have experienced many of the complications associated with C-section births. Haemorrhages complicated two of my births, a bladder trauma required me to have a urinary catheter for seven days, and I became anaemic after my haemorrhages. After one birth, I experienced post-traumatic stress disorder (PTSD). I needed medication for a premature labour, had a grade four placenta previa, and in two pregnancies developed gestational diabetes. With my sixth C-section, I developed placenta accreta and required an emergency hysterectomy. These experiences have both broadened and inspired my midwifery practice and passion for teaching.

I am indebted also to my nursing and midwifery colleagues, in particular, Jane Rose, Ali Rousseaux, Maree Kelly, Fiona Williams, Annette Garvey, Dr Kevin Rose, and Dr Hazel Keedle, for their encouragement and suggestions.

For the thousands of women I have supported through their surgery and hand-fashioned wound splints, thank you for trusting me. Thank you also to the women and couples who helped us truly understand their needs in terms of C-section preparation, education, and postpartum support.

We would also like to thank the publishers who encouraged us along the way and the reviewers who helped shape this book.

Finally, thank you to you the reader who has decided to explore all things C-section with us. We are honoured you want to have us along to support you on your journey to recovery.

Preface

As healthcare professionals, we have worked eighty-five years collectively in nursing and midwifery practice in maternity units, hospitals, and the community setting. Residing in the United Kingdom and Australia respectively, we first met at the inaugural International Maternity Expo in London in 2019. After discovering our shared passion for helping women through the transformative event that is birth, we decided to write a self-help recovery manual for women recovering from a C-section birth.

The reality of C-section birth and motherhood is one of the most challenging times in your life and a time to celebrate all the magic and relief of a safe birth. But real life is not like that, and the reason for needing a C-section in the first place can be your first challenge. Janine describes some journeys into motherhood as 'the car crash birth': an unsuccessful induction, an illness, assisted forceps or vacuum extraction birth that failed, an episiotomy, long labour that was unable to progress, a baby in distress, a low heartbeat, an ill mother, a mother haemorrhaging, a father waiting for news, women who develop sepsis, the mother with pre-eclampsia. These are just a few scenarios that, as midwives, we have seen in our careers. These women are our warriors. It is for all C-section women we wrote this manual—a legacy in the form of a virtual recovery manual, exploring the highs, the lows, the good, the bad, the joyful, and harrowing stories of the journeys some mothers experience as part of their journey into motherhood.

We have both observed mothers trying to navigate the emotional cocoon of motherhood after a C-section and experienced mothers trying to manage a range of issues including pain, fatigue, breastfeeding difficulties, lack of sleep, and dietary concerns. Many people do not understand that there is a whole-body recovery process from pregnancy to birth to postpartum.

The trend for shorter stays in the hospital following this major surgery and the need for well-informed self-care motivated us to create this manual. We could find little evidence of dedicated C-section education in antenatal classes. Based on questions posted on social media forums for C-section mothers, we have been able to identify the topics most needed to help bridge our identified knowledge gap.

Our project began as the global COVID-19 pandemic took hold, imposing travel and many other restrictions worldwide. Despite the physical distance between us, we have used online meetings and spent thousands of hours writing from the heart and current research to create this valuable resource.

Women need kindness and compassion during the transformative time following a C-section. We hope that both these values shine through our words as our desire is to honour and respect your birth experience and walk with you through the recovery period. Our intention is for this manual to act as a virtual midwife to enhance your recovery from C-section birth. *C-Section Recovery Manual: Your Body, Your Recovery* is not intended as a medical textbook; it is a C-section guide written by two nurses and midwives and is dedicated to supporting and equipping you for your recovery. Our aim is to answer your questions and concerns during your postpartum period and to help you understand the why, when, and how to manage your recovery period.

This book is for all women, for all the faces and journeys into motherhood, explicitly focusing on C-section birth and the realistic outcomes of achieving a positive postpartum recovery. We acknowledge and respect the mothers who go home without their baby; those who will always carry the scar of birth by C-section on their abdomen and need added emotional support during the postpartum period.

This manual is for all fathers, partners, and carers, too. You have also been strong, and you might seek inspiration and tools for how you can best support the new mother.

We hope that this C-section recovery manual will help you understand and appreciate the significant surgery you have been through and permit yourself to ease back into daily activities. Timely information and resources for women recovering from C-section can help mothers better enjoy bonding and attachment with their babies, free of pain, shame, or anxiety.

Our mission in co-writing this book is to inspire and equip women and their carers to experience an empowered, confident, and enjoyable recovery and transition into parenthood, and in return, achieve a sense of confidence in your own birthing story.

> C-section birth is definitely not the easy way out in my professional experience; in fact, apart from the convenience of being able to choose the date of birth, I think the inevitable pain associated and the mobility restrictions for the following six weeks make it far from easy!
>
> —Leonie Rastas

Introduction

An Australian television channel reported a powerful social media post by a new mother revealed she was cruelly shamed—and told she is not a 'real mother'—because she had a C-section instead of natural birth. Due to complications, she required a caesarean to save her and her baby's life potentially. The joy was soon dampened by an influx of comments—from relatives to strangers—that a C-section was the 'easy way out'.

The young mother also said, 'I had a nurse tell me to "get over" my pain, and that other women have it way worse because they gave birth naturally and "can't even sit down". I've had other people tell me that I've had the easy way out, that I didn't do anything, and just laid there. They told me I didn't give birth to my baby.'

Her post was acknowledged by hundreds of mothers who had also experienced backlash following a C-section birth, which the mother said showed how common this archaic sentiment is in 2020.[1]

This book will dispel those myths and give due respect to a significant surgery that is not the easy way out, especially given the impact C-section can have on a woman and the challenges during recovery.

Some typical comments and questions we, as healthcare providers, have heard after C-section birth, highlight how challenging C-section can be. For example: 'I am in so much pain I can't hold my baby,' 'Help me, I am bleeding,' and 'I am scared'. 'When can I have another baby?' 'Will I be able to have a baby vaginally next time?' 'How do I breastfeed?' 'I am passing blood clots. Is this normal?' 'Why did I have a C-section?' or, 'I am not bonding with my baby.'

C-Section Recovery Manual: Your Body, Your Recovery is written about navigating the C-section journey from preparation through to the end of the six-week recovery period, also known as the postpartum period. The International Confederation of Midwives (ICM), in its core document on the philosophy and model of midwifery care, states that:

> Midwives provide women with appropriate information and advice in a way that promotes participation and enhances informed decision-making. [and] Midwives empower women to assume responsibility for their health and their families' health.[2]

We intend that this book will achieve both of these goals for women who have C-section births.

The impact of the COVID-19 global pandemic is seeing women being forced to birth without partner support and spending less time in hospital receiving midwifery care.[3] Now is the time to empower women and their partners and carers with knowledge and skills to self-manage their recovery. Our manual is designed to do just that. We consider the global experiences of women having C-sections in our manual and hope to provide added support particularly for women who face early discharge from hospital. The 2019 OECD indicators report caesarean section rates vary from 15%–17% in the Nordic countries to 45%–53% in Korea, Chile, Mexico, and Turkey.[4] In the United Kingdom, where Janine is based and has over forty-two years of maternity nursing care practice, 27.4% of women will birth by C-section, while in Australia, the OECD reports 32.5% of women will have a C-section birth.[5] Between their global combined career of eighty-five years, both have achieved an award-winning career in this field. Both are passionate about improving the recovery knowledge and resources available to C-section women.

C-Section Recovery Manual: Your Body, Your Recovery addresses the fears and uncertainty many women face relating to C-section: fears such as those highlighted earlier, and concerns about scar healing, returning to regular activity, fatigue, and other preventative postoperative challenges. The book is written in the form of a three-part manual to guide you through the postpartum:

- Part One will provide you with explanations and twelve chapters dedicated to the significant challenges that C-section women can experience.
- Part Two contains blank journal pages to help you and process your thoughts and feelings using words, drawings, or photographs.
- Part Three consists of daily planners and a scar tracker guide to help keep track of wound healing, medications, remind you of essential self-care steps, and record milestones during your postpartum recovery. Appendices are also included in Part Three: the birth plan, the daily planner, the scar tracker, gift suggestions, and tips on managing constipation.

We trust you will find valuable information in our manual and feel empowered to move through the healing process armed with your very own virtual midwife manual to support and encourage you.

We wish you well with your birth journey and hope you enjoy this book as a helpful daily companion on your recovery journey.

Just a mention, too, for your birth partners, husband, partner, boyfriend, girlfriend, or wife—this manual can help you to help them understand your special needs.

References

1. Seven News, *So disheartening': Adelaide mum shamed on social media after giving birth via C-section,* 2019, viewed June 2021, https://7news.com.au/lifestyle/so-disheartening-adelaide-mum-shamed-on-social-media-after-giving-birth-via-c-section--c-1250575.

2. International Confederation of Midwives, *Philosophy and Model of Midwifery Care*, 2014, viewed June 2021, https://www.internationalmidwives.org/assets/files/general-files/2020/07/cd0005_v201406_en_philosophy-and-model-of-midwifery-care.pdf.

3. CBS News, *Pregnant women are forced to give birth alone as hospitals restrict visitors during coronavirus,* 2020, viewed June 2021, https://www.cbsnews.com/news/coronavirus-pregnant-women-hospitals-give-birth-alone/

4. Organisation for Economic Cooperation and Development, *Caesarean sections,* OECD, 2019, viewed June 2021, https://www.oecd-ilibrary.org/sites/fa1f7281-en/index.html?itemId=/content/component/fa1f7281-en

5. NHS Digital, *Maternity Services Monthly Statistics January 2019, Experimental Statistics,* July 2019, viewed June 2021, https://digital.nhs.uk/data-and-information/publications/statistical/maternity-services-monthly-statistics/january-2019

Part One

Understanding Caesarean Section Birth

Chapter 1
What is a caesarean section birth?

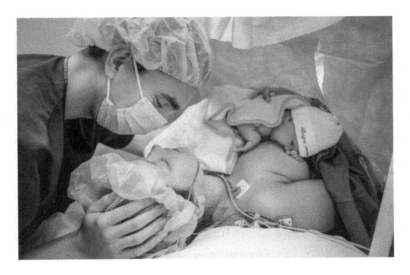

A caesarean section is an operation in which a baby is born through an incision (cut) made through the women's abdomen and the uterus (womb). The cut is usually made low and around the level of the bikini line. A caesarean section may be planned (elective) if there is a reason that prevents the baby from being born by a normal vaginal birth, or unplanned (emergency) if complications develop and birth needs to be quick. This may be before or during your labour.

The history of the caesarean section

The exact origin of the term *caesarean* is not clear; artworks from ancient Roman times suggest caesarean birth was performed during that era. However, some say it was named later after the surgical birth of Julius Caesar.

Perhaps the first written record we have of a mother and baby surviving a caesarean section comes from Switzerland in 1500, when a sow gelder, Jacob Nufer, operated on his wife. After several days in labour and help from thirteen midwives, the woman could not deliver her baby, so he went ahead and performed the surgery.[6]

A study by Katz et al. published by the journal *Obstetrics & Gynecology* in 1995 believed a review in terminology was needed and the term 'cesarean section' should be abandoned, reporting it had recently been amended to 'cesarean birth'.[7] It is interesting to note the peak bodies in the Colleges of Obstetricians and Gynaecologists in the UK and Australia still use 'caesarean section' terminology whilst the USA refer to 'cesarean births'. The recommendation from the 1995 study suggested the term 'hysterotomy' be a preferable adjective to describe the procedure, *hyster* being Latin for uterus and -*otomy* a suffix meaning a surgical cutting into part of the body. The authors recommended the following new terms for caesarean births: 'classical hysterotomy' for the vertical incision, 'contemporary hysterotomy' for the low transverse caesarean, 'neoclassical hysterotomy' for a low vertical procedure, and 'transitional hysterotomy' for the 'hockey stick' or 'J' incision. The study also recommended that vaginal birth after hysterotomy (VBAH) should become a substitute for VBAC. I guess we have held onto the 'caesarean section' terminology for 520 years, so it may be some time before we warm to the new language proposed twenty-five years ago!

Carley's story

Induction had never been discussed until I reached forty weeks.

The disappointment I felt is unmatched to this day—a huge bleed resulting from so much intervention, fatigue, and faltering heartbeats in my sons' recordings. Almost three full days of intervention led to an emergency section. During the C-section, they found my placenta had torn from my uterus. My disappointment was met with a thankfulness that my son was, in a sense, rescued. I found strength through allowing myself to heal, as cliché as it may sound, I knew I had endured and given it my best shot.

Why do women have C-sections?

There are multiple reasons women have C-sections, ranging from medically indicated, to emergency, to mother's choice—often referred to as maternal request caesarean section (MRCS). The C-section birth option can be scheduled for personal reasons as a maternal choice; C-section birth can be life-saving for both you and the baby when medically indicated.

Whatever the reason, it will be a life-changing event for a mother. Over our lifetime, we accumulate life experiences, pregnancy, birth, and motherhood that are identifiable as life-changing events. Paying full attention to ourselves, both good and bad, involves a whole new human being. The spiritual and emotional dynamic between mother and child is important. We have seen mothers putting themselves last at a time where they should be the priority—often choosing to still do washing, cooking, cleaning, shopping, and household chores as opposed to resting and recuperating and bonding with their babies.

The social, economic acceptance of C-sections in many countries, coupled with the fact that women today are spending less and less time in the hospital, makes paying proper attention to the major surgery experience you have just gone through all the more critical.

A strategy for self-management of wound-healing—and generally, a holistic approach to your whole wellbeing—is imperative.

Education and the practice of mindfulness in recognising feelings, signs, and symptoms cultivate who you are and help you identify with yourself. In many cultures, it is customary for extra women—the mother-in-law or the woman's mother or sister, for example—to attend the birth. Some women who have migrated to Australia from other cultures find it distressing that this custom is not the norm. Women are often well-supported by the extended family during the postpartum period in many cultures also.[8] In Australia's First Nations people, the social organisation of kinship can provide birthing women with a supportive environment, but this is not always available.

Developing a mindset where you put yourself at the centre of your recovery from day one through the six weeks of the postpartum period will help enhance your recovery. Building in self-reflective time to focus on your physical, mental, and spiritual wellbeing will help guide your journey and make wise choices also.

Why do women have C-sections?
Maternal Reasons
Previous C-sections, Placenta Praevia, Maternal Choice, Medical conditions, Placental abruption, Previous birth trauma, HIV, Herpes, Blood disorders.

Baby Reasons
Baby lying sideways, Breech with feet first, Twin pregnancy with breech first, Multiple pregnancies, Some congenital abnormalities, Prematurity or growth.

Emergency Reasons
Antenatal haemorrhage, Uterine rupture, Pre-eclampsia, HELLP syndrome, Obstructed Labour, Baby at risk, Cord prolapse, Fetal (baby) distress.

How is a C-section performed?
A spinal/epidural or general anaesthetic will be administered as preparation for surgery. The doctor will use a scalpel blade to make a horizontal or vertical incision into your skin and the layers below. The most common incision is the horizontal type just above the pubic bone and under the bikini line. Some women may get a vertical midline incision cut if required for medical reasons.

Once the skin, fat layer, muscle, and peritoneum are opened, a cut through into the uterus or womb allows the surgeon to reach your baby.

The fluid-filled amniotic sac surrounding the baby will be ruptured, followed by your baby being lifted out by your surgeon. Sometimes forceps may be needed to lift the baby's head if its head is lodged deep into the pelvic cradle. The umbilical cord is cut once the cord stops pulsating, and then, if all is well, the baby is wrapped and is placed on your chest, providing there are no breathing or health issues.

The surgeon will then remove your baby's placenta, after which they will fully repair the uterine, peritoneal, muscle, fat, and skin layers. They will close the skin using clips, stitches, glue, or wound closure strips, and the skin wound is protected with an appropriate surgical dressing.

The baby will then be weighed, their length measured, and a full physical examination will usually be performed in the recovery room. You will typically spend around sixty minutes in the operating room for a C-section, depending upon whether any complications arise during the birth. Following surgery, you will spend time in the operating department's recovery room to ensure your vital signs are stable before you go to the postnatal ward.

What are the advantages, disadvantages, and potential risks of a C-section birth?

It is essential to know and understand what is involved in the surgery to enable you to make an informed decision. Your birth partner could also be the one to help support you make this decision, so this is worth sharing. Caesarean section involves many decisions before you even reach the operating theatre. Preparation is the key and understanding the procedure will help you manage your recovery. A C-section birth plan is worth considering, helping you consider the experience you want or might receive due to an emergency.[9]

Mother

Advantages	Disadvantages (potential risks)
Predictability	Post-surgery weakness, fatigue
No labour pains	Extended hospital stay
No injury to the vagina	Potential uterus infection
Lower risk of urinary incontinence	Bowel or bladder injury
Lower risk of vaginal prolapse	Possible delay establishing breastfeeding
Convenience	Harder to look after the baby
Shorter birthtime	Unable to drive for 4–6 weeks
	Clinical setting surrounded by strangers
	Future placental abnormalities/uterine rupture
	Limited in activity and weights to be lifted
	Wound pain/infection/separation
	Clothing restrictions
	Slower to return to exercise
	Thromboembolic disease
	Anaesthetic complications
	Potential future fertility issues

Baby

Advantages	Disadvantages (potential risks)
	Breathing difficulties, asthma, obesity in children
	Higher risk of admission to the neonatal unit
	Skin laceration, organ damage, and infection

RCOG; 2009 retrieved from https://www.rcog.org.uk/globalassets/documents/guidelines/consent-advice/ca7-15072010.pdf.

Figure 1.1 Advantages and Disadvantages C-section

L Rastas (2020)

What will happen on the day the C-section is scheduled?

Planned C-section schedule

Each country and hospital will have its own guidance and established service offering. This is intended to be a guide on what to expect. In an emergency, this schedule will change depending upon the degree of risk.

Preparation for surgery

Fasting from food and fluid for six hours prior to birth is important in order to avoid complications should you vomit during surgery.

Assessments

Your midwife and anaesthetic nurse will need to assess all your vital signs, and baby's position and heart rate, before surgery. A urine sample will also be taken for testing.

Transport to theatre

In some facilities, you will be able to walk to the operating theatre as a means of creating more normality around the birth. In other facilities, transport will be via a hospital bed or transport trolley. In an emergency, it is likely you will be transferred in your hospital bed.

Intravenous drip

A general, epidural, or spinal anaesthetic procedure will require you to have an intravenous catheter (IV, or 'drip') inserted into the back of your hand/arm. This will be to allow intravenous fluids to support you during surgery. It will be removed once you are eating and drinking again, usually within a few hours of birth.

Urinary catheter

It is vital that the bladder be empty during surgery to reduce the risk of bladder injury from the scalpel, so a catheter will be inserted and attached to a drainage bag. The catheter will remain in place until the next day and be removed once you are confident walking and eating and drinking well. This is very helpful, as during the first twenty-four hours, a large volume of fluid passes after the IV fluids in theatre, so it saves a lot of trips to the bathroom.

Antacid medication

You may also be required to drink an antacid preparation to help neutralise stomach acid and reduce risks in case of vomiting during surgery.

Compression stockings

Anti-embolism stockings help to keep blood moving back to the heart rather than pooling in the lower limbs and forming clots, leading to serious consequences from deep vein thrombosis (DVT).

Theatre gown and cap

A special theatre gown will be issued. If wishing to breastfeed in theatre of the recovery room, it is a good idea to ask if you can wear the gown with the opening to the front for easy breast access for both mother and baby.

Make-up and vail varnish

Any nail varnish or jewellery items may need to be removed depending on hospital policy. The fingertips give a good gauge as to the status of circulation and are a useful guide, however, technology is now able to assess circulation status with oximeter probes.

Partner or support person attire

Surgical caps are required, and your birth partner or support person will also need to be prepared and changed into theatre clothing before joining you in the operating room.

Setting up your hospital room

If admitted to your room before the baby's birth, it's a good idea to try to unpack your items to include lip balm, chewing gum (known for its bowel stimulant properties), hand-wipes, tissues, notepad, and pen, wound splint, or pillow. Have these within easy reach as, initially, you will be limited in your movement on returning to your room.

Mindset

Do whatever works for you to be in a calm and relaxed state before being transferred to the theatre. Some women prefer to listen to music, others to meditate or pray; find what works best for you. Just as childbirth's physical experience is different for every woman so, too, is their spiritual experience. For women who prefer a quiet, low-lit space for birth, creating a calm and sacred space is not easy in a sterile operating theatre packed with machines and bright lights. Playing soothing music with earphones may be right for you, or using essential oils, eyeshades, breathing exercises, and visualisation or meditation on calming spiritual images that speak to you individually. Remember, your right to embrace your spiritual practices during this life-changing time should be respected. What may seem irrational to others should not diminish your resolve to attend to your spiritual wishes during this time. Just as in vaginal birth, couples should prepare their space and feel safe and respected in their zone physically, emotionally, and spiritually. So, too, should you, remembering, of course, that safety in the operating theatre is paramount. You should be able to create the space you desire once you return to your hospital room, e.g., dim lighting, music, quiet time together. It is vital to draw on all your resources and power during the birth of your precious baby.

Anaesthesia

The anaesthetist will discuss appropriate anaesthesia with you, and the choice will depend on the given situation for the C-section. General anaesthetic requires a sedation that will mean you are fully asleep. Spinal anaesthesia will allow you to be awake but have no nerve feeling from mid-abdomen to toes. Consent to proceed will be required, and in some complications, a spinal can proceed to a general anaesthetic.

Intravenous drip and urinary catheter

Before surgery, your doctor/midwife will insert a urinary catheter into your bladder and connect it to a drainage bag to keep your bladder empty for the next twelve to twenty-four hours—a safety procedure and support for you in the early hours after birth. As you have an intravenous infusion, you will expect to make a lot of urine, but you won't get the sensation to urinate if you have had a spinal anaesthetic.

In the operating theatre

There will be a team of staff in the theatre, so be prepared for all the new faces. In addition to your surgeon and assistant, there will be an anaesthetist, a paediatrician, a midwife, theatre nurses, a theatre technician. You may also have a professional photographer in addition to your partner. Safety is the key. Who gets to attend will be decided by the surgeon; a formal request is often made if a photographer is requested.

The C-section process

Surgical drapes are positioned in front of your chest to obscure your view of surgery. These can be lowered if you want to see your baby lifted out.

After the uterus opening is made and before the baby is birthed, you will likely experience pulling and tugging sensations as the doctor makes the incision wide enough for the baby; however, this should not register as pain. If, by chance, you experience pain, let your anaesthetist know straight away so action can be taken to support you.

After baby and the placenta are delivered

Paediatric care is provided to check your baby once it is born. The baby's care at birth will affect whether immediate skin-to-skin or chest to your chest contact will be safe. Skin to skin is beneficial for many reasons to enhance attachment and bonding and support breastfeeding's biological responses.

The surgeon will repair your abdomen using internal stitches and staples or surgical wound adhesives, and you will eventually be relocated to the recovery room for a period of observation. During this time, if you and your baby are well enough, there can be an opportunity to try breastfeeding.

If you plan more children, when the surgeon is finalising your stitching is a good time to ask your doctor if your uterus is in good condition.

Post-operative recovery

You will spend some time in a special observation area after leaving theatre and before returning to your room. Here your vital signs, wound, vaginal loss, and pain score will be assessed. After you leave the recovery room, you will be transferred to your post-natal room, usually thirty-sixty minutes after birth.

Resuming food and fluids

On your return to the ward, you will probably begin oral fluid intake again, starting with ice chips to suck and a little while later, fluids and food. You will be able to eat and drink when you feel up to it and any nausea or vomiting has abated. A diet high in fibre and multivitamins will enhance healing and help avoid constipation.

Pain relief

The stretching and internal bruising, along with the incision's tenderness, are the primary sources of postoperative pain. It's important to take regular medication to control that pain. While you will not be pain-free in the early days, the medicine and other supportive treatments like a cold pack application should keep you comfortable. You may experience afterbirth pains if this is your second baby, especially during breastfeeding, as the uterus contracts to expel the blood. Maintaining a daily recovery planner (Part Three) will allow you to track your recovery, pain, and general wellbeing.

Monitoring

Your blood pressure, pulse, temperature, vaginal blood loss, and wound will be checked regularly in the first twelve to twenty-four hours after surgery, then recorded up to three times per day while still in the hospital.

Your wound will be checked regularly for bleeding, bruising, or swelling. Protecting your injury with a cushion, rolled towel, or dedicated splint is essential to avoid unnecessary pain and potential breaking of stitches during sudden movements such as coughing, sneezing, or laughing.

Bladder and bowels

The urinary catheter is removed when you are drinking well and able to walk to the bathroom. Urine output will need to be measured and observed for early detection of any bladder dysfunction. Maintaining a daily recovery planner (Part Three) will allow you to track your recovery, pain, and general wellbeing.

Visitors

A point to remember is that while you may feel excellent and well enough for visitors on the same day, C-section is major surgery. Many women become overwhelmed by excited visitors on day one, so do consider conserving your energy for at least twenty-four hours. You will be glad you did.

Self-care/hygiene

The first shower is amazingly soothing, so don't be reluctant. The effect of hot water on the skin is heavenly. Get your partner or midwife to help dry your back initially. Avoid attempting your first shower on your own. Fainting is a common problem after surgery. Ask for help if you need it.

Feeding baby

Whether breast or bottle feeding, you will need assistance to position the baby to not apply pressure on the wound. Mastering the art of side-lying feeding in bed is helpful. Maintaining a daily recovery planner (Part Three) will allow you to track your baby's feeding and waking times.

Sleep

Getting comfortable in the first few days is difficult, so be sure to keep up with your pain-relief regime. It's not wise to skip a dose as peaks in pain will be unpleasant. A pillow at your back and another between the knees could be helpful.

Baby care

It is ideal to have your partner stay for the first night at least, as it is challenging to lift your baby in the early few days; if you don't have your partner or a friend able to stay, buzz your midwife to help.

It can help place nappies and wipes on a surface at waist height to save unnecessary bending.

Be sure to have bed rails up when alone with the baby as it is easy to fall asleep holding the baby and lose your grip. It is especially important to avoid accidentally dropping the baby when taking pain relief in the early days, or post-general anaesthetic.

Summary

The birth of a baby is a momentous occasion in anyone's life. A C-section birth can invoke emotions of fear, shame, guilt, and anxiety which can compete with joy and excitement. These emotions can also interfere with bonding and attachment with the baby. Dealing with worries and fears when preparing for C-section will help prevent these feelings. Fear of the unknown is a significant contributor to anxiety, so asking questions and seeking information from your healthcare providers can reduce the impact of worries.

Having a clear idea of the schedule on the day of your surgery should also help. Ideally, a tour of the hospital and theatre area can help you visualise and personalise your experience in theatre and make it feel less clinical; check out what is possible at your hospital. While emergency C-sections don't always allow time to create such environments, the experience can still be profoundly personal and uplifting.

All C-section births call for bravery and strength to have major surgery whilst fully awake and then afterward to cope with the limitations during the recovery period. Be proud of yourself and don't let anyone tell you took the easy way out; you will know the fatigue and limitations that follow major surgery only too well, so believe in yourself and be proud, strong, and confident of the fact that what you have experienced takes fierce courage and strength!

References

6. US National Library of Medicine, *Caesarean section - A Brief History,* USNLM, 2013, viewed June 2021, https://www.nlm.nih.gov/exhibition/cesarean/part1.html.

7. V L Katz, et al., 'Cesarean delivery: a reconsideration of terminology', *Obstetrics & Gynecology,* vol. 86, issue 1, pp. 152-153, viewed June 2021, https://pubmed.ncbi.nlm.nih.gov/7784013/.

8. N Boules, *Cultural Birthing Practices and Experiences,* Baulkham Hills Holroyd Parramatta Migrant Resource Centre, viewed June 2021, https://cmrc.com.au/wp-content/uploads/2020/03/cultural_birthing_practices_and_experiences.pdf.

9. Royal Australian and New Zealand College of Obstetricians and Gynaecologists, *Caesarean Section,* RANZCOG, 2019, viewed June 2021, https://ranzcog.edu.au/womens-health/patient-information-resources/caesarean-section; C Nierenberg, *Vaginal Birth vs.C-section:Pros & Cons,* Future US, 2018, viewed https://www.livescience.com/45681-vaginal-birth-vs-c-section.html.

Chapter 2
Five Guide—a tool to support your understanding of C-sections

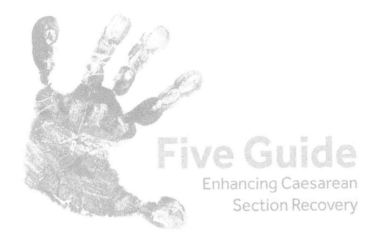

Figure 2.1 Five Guide

https://rcni.com/primary-health-care/features/simple-visual-tool-helps-safeguard-mothers-after-caesarean-section-150506[10]

Keeley's story

Five Guide helped us all after the birth of my fourth baby. My previous section was with my twins fifteen years previously. At this section, we all knew what to expect, who could help, and what my older children could do to support me. I realised the pain was so deeply felt because I thought of my muscles and my womb healing, instead of relying on looking at my bruised and scar tissue for answers. Hoovering, washing, and cooking support all came much easier to my team of helpers, as they all understood the surgery I'd had and just how long it was going to take me to recover. Five Guide is a mother's help tool; I think all mothers should know about it.

In this chapter, we can combine the theory and knowledge with a visual explanation of why recovery matters. One of the reasons the caesarean section recovery innovation 'Five Guide' has become so popular with women who have had a C-section is that it explains in a straightforward visual narrative:

- What is a C-section?
- What has happened to me?
- How will I heal?
- The five anatomical layers which will be healing.
- How to use the scar tracker to observe your wound healing (see Appendix 3 in Part Three).

Quite simply: Five Guide is the 3D explanation of our five-layer abdominal healing process. We are raising your awareness to the repair internally behind that bikini-line skin surgical incision. Janine created Five Guide, and it has developed it into an award-winning and clinically significant post-C-section recovery tool.[10]

As a midwife, Janine discussed wound healing with clients and, in her experience, she felt that women appear to believe the skin and bikini line scar is the only part of their abdomen healing. This led to the development of Five Guide as a visual explanation. The video will help you and your support network to see and understand your surgery. Whilst developing and using Five Guide in practice, Janine discovered the benefits of talking in layman's terms on what a mother might find beneficial in understanding her physical and emotional symptoms.

Five Guide allows women to know how much is healing, where, and why it takes so long to recover.

It would be good at this point to view the Five Guide video. This will give you a visual opportunity to understand what your surgery involves, see what happens in a surgical view inside your body, and see the five layers that need to heal.

Take a break, pop the book down, and check out the YouTube video. Follow the link below.

Figure 2.2 Five guide
<https://www.youtube.com/watch?v=EwbLFdjHH_0>
This work was developed by Janine as part of her research and innovation award.

The essential functions of our 'autopilot' controls in life will now require our full attention. A sharp abdominal pain abruptly reminds you of your inability to simply reach across the bed to drink a glass of water; it is a reminder that you had surgery, a reminder that you need to take pain relief.

Finally, a reminder that there is also a baby who needs you. The power of patterns, reactions, feelings, and behaviour are all linked.

These links can also be understood by using your daily planners (Part Three). Simple routines postpartum help to build your reflective resilience to pain management, diet, rest, etc., in order to support healing and recovery. They will also enhance bonding and attachment as each item on the daily planner is designed to link the why, when, and how you make choices to support your daily recovery.

What is Five Guide?

Five Guide is a visual tool for women, their families, and health professionals. It uses the hand and its five digits to explain the five abdominal layers of healing involved after a C-section.

How does it work?

The hand is used, held high with five fingers spread. Each finger from thumb to a small finger is a visual window of internal healing. Visualising your abdominal healing from the outer skin to the inner womb in five layers reinforces your healing process. Each digit represents a healing abdominal layer as follows:

Layer 1—Thumb

There are several incisions an obstetrician can make. The most common is a horizontal 'bikini' incision in the lower skin abdomen.

Layer 2—Index finger

A smaller tract of cutting then takes place through the fat layer.

Layer 3—Middle finger

The rectus abdominal muscles (the abs) are two muscles that run from the upper abdomen down to the pubic bone. Where they meet can easily be separated with a gentle pushing away at the midline to expose the next layer to open.

Layer 4—Ring finger

The next layer is the peritoneum, a thin film that is the actual lining of the abdomen.

Layer 5—Little finger

The abdominal cavity is opened very carefully with scissors. It is so thin you can see the bowel and bladder through it. A retractor is inserted to protect other organs from getting in the way. The uterus or (womb) is then fully exposed and covered in another peritoneum layer over it. With the uterus exposed and the bladder protected, the womb is now available to proceed to birth.

Closing the C-section wound in reverse order

The value of understanding your surgical birth can support you in your recovery. Once your baby is born, the placenta or afterbirth is delivered manually from the uterine wall.

By the time everyone is waiting for the baby to cry, the surgeon has tilted the womb through all the incisions made and has then laid it onto the mother's abdomen for easy access to begin suturing back together in layers, and in reverse:

Layer 5—Little finger
The uterine wall will be the first layer to be sewn together, closing off vessels and reducing bleeding following delivery.

Layer 4—Ring finger
The peritoneum will be drawn back together and will heal and close on its own.

Layer 3—Middle finger
The abdominal muscles start to come back together and, in some cases, can heal by themselves. Some surgeons may gently tie them together at spots along their length. Fascia repair containing the abdominal organs needs a more durable repair.

Layer 2—Index finger
The fat layer can also come together with isolated absorbable sutures.

Layer 1—Thumb
The skin, the weakest of the whole five-layer repair, is gently brought together and either stitched, glued, stapled, or drawn together with sterile adhesive tapes.

**Five Guide
is an innovative
visual tool to enhance
caesarean section recovery.**

Five Guide is a nurse developed commitment to Better Births for all.

A visual health promotion tool to use with women who have caesarean section.

Five Guide is the visual narrative of our anatomy that improves womens knowledge and understanding of the five layer healing process.

These are:

1. Skin > 2. Fat > 3. Muscle > 4. Peritoneum > 5. Womb

Five layers could take up to 5-6 weeks to heal.

Clinicians using just their hand as a visual symbol engages women in their own internal healing process. Inspiring all who care for surgically delivered women to use a consistent and sustainable tool.

For more information please contact
Janine McKnight-Cowan on janinemcknight@nhs.net

 youtu.be/EwbLFdjHH_0

Supported by

 RCN Foundation

The Healing Process

As the coming hours, days, and weeks progress, you will begin to see, feel, and take part in your recovery journey. Those around you whom you have chosen as your support network can be shown the Five Guide video in order to support their nurturing and realistic understanding of your needs. Developing and building on your daily planners and journal entries (Parts Two and Three) will also give you a reflective log to record and see your progress.

The excitement of this new little miracle—your baby—joining you in your home is welcomed and celebrated. Along with a welcome celebration of the baby, let there be planning and promotion of the mother's recovery.

Consider how your new baby's whole day is planned, from what cute garment they wear, to nursing and feeding, if we let them cry or if we just stare and gaze at them, it is all about protection, feeding, and nurturing.

Reasonable care should include the nurturing and care of two people: mother and baby.

Self-preservation is not a selfish act; it is a continuation of the postpartum maintenance required to recover following surgical birth.

In fact, as a midwife, I always focused upon the mother and father's coping mechanisms on the first home visit—usually on day three to day fourteen post-birth. If parents appeared relaxed, cared for, and under no additional stress, the baby was less likely to be crying, underfed, or experiencing its difficulties because its parents could not pick up on its cues due to their own unmet needs.

The impact of Five Guide on enhancing recovery

When Five Guide was introduced into general practice, some fantastic new outcomes were achieved:

- The educational tool helped fathers and partners to understand the importance of facilitating internal recovery. This led to all-important shared choices relating to birth control, rest, dietary needs, medication needs, recovery, sleep, maternal wellbeing, physical strength, and sexual relationships.
- Five Guide, as a tool, creates the perfect opportunity to engage with women in a personal response to the surgery and experience they have been through, opening up the debriefing discussions which may identify unresolved anxieties relating to the birth.
- Practically, an improved visual understanding of the physical anatomy, and the need (*why*) to enhance knowledge, can support you with pain relief (*what* you can do to relieve symptoms), highlighting the need to engage your support networks (*how*) so, in turn, others can support you in areas of household chores, meal preparation, and other recovery needs.

Women reported to us the straightforward visual narrative was consistent and sustainable when measuring pain and physical ability, thus quickly equipping them with the ability to understand their pain or injury.

As an innovative resource, the Five Guide tool has won national awards for innovative practice.

Janine was invited to present Five Guide at the Inaugural International Maternity Expo in London in 2019 where she first met co-author Leonie and the idea of writing this manual was conceived. You could even say it was the time that conceiving the *C-section Recovery Manual: Your Body, Your Recovery* occurred.

Five Guide as a recovery tool allows the simple anatomical explanation of why 'taking it easy' after abdominal surgery is necessary, not a luxury.

Scar tracker—keeping an eye on your wound

The scar tracker (Appendix 1 in Part Three) is designed to help you know what to look for on a daily basis as your scar heals. Early detection of breakdown and infection is vital to ensure timely treatment for best outcomes and to avoid delays in healing. Be sure to make a habit of viewing your incision line daily and note your findings on your scar tracker. If you don't have a floor-length mirror in a well-lit area, it will be wise to take a hand-held mirror and move into a better-lit area. Your doctor usually doesn't see your scar again until the six-week check-up, so it's up to you to monitor its progress and seek medical advice if any of the symptoms or signs listed on the tracker appear.

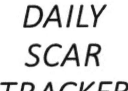

DAILY SCAR TRACKER

30 Day Scar Tracker

Describe your scar and decide if you need a review

1	2	3
4	5	6
7	8	9
10	11	12
13	14	15
16	17	18
19	20	21
22	23	24
25	26	27
28	29	30

Normal pattern of healing

- Clean dry, pink/red suture line
- No swelling, pain, minor fluid loss
- No fever, no odour, no swelling
- Pain score reducing
- Possibly some wound itching

Abnormal Signs and Symptoms

- Fever
- Wound is hot, red, and painful
- Wound is oozing copious fluids
- An offensive odour from wound

If you experience abnormal signs and symptoms: SEEK MEDICAL REVIEW

Use this Scar Tracker to view, record, and decide on what to do if you suspect your wound is not healing as well as you would expect. Use the indicators above to record in the day tracker your findings. Seek medical opinion if you suspect a wound infection or breakdown. It is easier to use a hand-held mirror to observe your wound. Some wound dressings are time specific in their removal.

Appendix 1

Seek medical advice if any of the symptoms or signs listed on the tracker appear.[11]

Summary

This chapter has explored an essential and important early topic. Without knowing 'what is a C-section' and 'Five Guide,' you, the reader, the mother, the partner, or support person would not make fully informed decisions. Decisions are needed for the coming days and weeks ahead, as well as decisions on future pregnancies and birth methods. Keeping an eye on your scar as it heals is also essential for you to get help if you feel you need it. The Scar tracker helps identify any symptoms or signs you must be aware of.

As we progress through each new chapter of *Your Body, Your Recovery*, we will build your independence, knowledge, and information so you can be the mother you want to be, your support network can help you, and you can have a positive recovery plan.

References

10. J McKnight-Cowan, *Five Guide,* Royal College of Nursing, 2019, viewed June 2021, via https://rcni.com/primary-health-care/features/simple-visual-tool-helps-safeguard-mothers-after-caesarean-section-150506.

11. Rastas, L.M, McKnight-Cowan, J. (2022) Scar Tracker. https://bit.ly/3GSn11V

Chapter 3
The birth debrief—why is it so helpful?

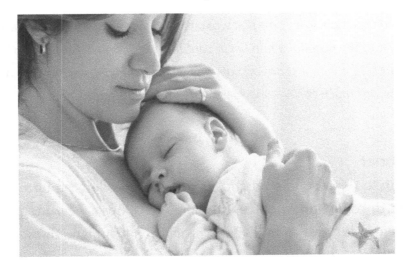

Why you should read this chapter:

- To understand that reflection is an encouraging process to understand what happened to you and why.
- To be aware of your spiritual wellbeing postoperatively.
- To explore the prevalence of post-birth psychological trauma.
- To be able to contribute to your reproductive health and decision-making in the future.

Sophie's story

My first birth was an emergency C-section, and a traumatic one at that. It took me a while to even contemplate going through delivery again. Gradually, though, the memories do fade (not disappear) and the desire to have a sibling for my daughter made me decide I could do it. I went for a consultant appointment and made the decision to have a planned C-section this time; I couldn't face going through the long-drawn-out pain again and panicked at the idea of having a second emergency event. My second daughter had other plans and arrived vaginally two hours before my planned C-section. Whilst my first was a forty-two-hour labour, this time we only just made it to the hospital. I had never contemplated vaginal birth after C-section (VBAC), but I did it with just gas and air, and I'm so glad I did, because the recovery afterwards was much easier, especially with a three-year-old at home!

The birth debrief

An introduction to this valuable practice is something called the birth debrief. Birth debrief—or birth reflection opportunity—aims to allow a new mother to discuss her birth experience with a midwifery professional and minimise any adverse psychological effects.

It's just over three years since the *Better Births* report was published, referred to as a 'Five Year Forward View' for UK maternity services. Developed alongside the review of other public services, *Better Births* included the complete review of maternity services for women in the UK, including the offer of continuity of carer.[12] This means the same midwife overseeing antenatal care and postnatal care. However, in reality, the review provided opportunities for the women's needs to be heard. Women's needs were listened to and acted upon.

Part of twenty-first-century health service challenges means there are widespread views on what is needed. Activists like the National Childbirth Trust want clinically significant services. They offer quality care that is humane, respectful, involving, and empowering—addressing not only the medical model of care but also the tension between risk reduction and a social model of care. A social model of care includes mind, body, and spiritual care, ensuring birth debriefing is holistic and made available to every mother. You need to be able to discuss issues that affect you. Even if it leads to a complaint (or legal action), all women require that choice.

Australian maternity services are a mix of public and private facilities with planning and birth protocol predominantly undertaken by the states and territories through publicly funded programs and the Commonwealth. Australian maternity services encompass eleven different models of care. There are currently no consistent directives in postnatal services to offer debriefing after birth; therefore, not all women will have the opportunity through their experience.[13]

Midwives and other healthcare professionals who offer women the opportunity to talk about their childbirth experience should ideally and clearly describe the purpose. As midwives, we have always encouraged women to 'tell their birth story' at the first home visit following birth.

In conversation, women are allowed to tell their whole story—all the good and anything that had been upsetting. During our careers, we have found that debriefing forms the basis of assessing needs and helps shape the individual therapeutic care plan. For some women, it can be about the positive. Still, for most women, it has often reflected and opened the opportunity to stop, look back, focus on sensations and interventions: the *why*, *what*, and *how* things happened on the day. Spending whatever time it takes to allow the mind to focus allows you as a new mother and her partner to look back on what you have just experienced.

An example of birth debriefing: we recently asked a question on Facebook group 'Caesarean Section Support Australia & New Zealand', *What would you want to know more about following your C-section?*

An overwhelming response always seemed to come right back at us when opening the opportunity to discuss the birth. When we recently enquired about mothers' experiences of birth debriefing through a Facebook poll for the purposes of writing this chapter, it amazed us how many questions were shared, only serving to highlight the lost opportunity these women had experienced in not having a formal debrief. It alarmed us to think of how many unresolved issues and unanswered questions these women were left with and the potential impact on their mental health and wellbeing. Unresolved grief, anger, judgment, anxiety, depression, and stress could well surface without the debrief experience.

Some of the unresolved issues that were exposed within debriefing raised the hairs on the back of our necks. Responding to the women's concerns provided inspiration for the shape and design of our manual.

What, *why*, and *how* knowledge-sharing and questions can lead you to explore any unresolved issues. The format we employ in the manual attempts to pre-empt and include a range of possible postoperative experiences.

We believe that every woman in every country would benefit from a birth debrief. It lays the foundation for their recovery. Fathers and birth partners also need an opportunity to birth debrief, especially if they have been traumatised by what they saw, heard, and experienced as a birth partner.

Here is a selection of what questions came back to us on the Facebook poll; you'll see what we mean.

Facebook Question – *What would you want to know more about following your C-section?*

Q. I had the baby a week ago—why do I still have swollen feet?
A. Swollen feet occur due to oedema, or body fluid build-up in the veins in the legs after pregnancy. Try mobilising a little by walking, and rest your legs raised on a footstool.

Q. Why did my whole body shake after the birth?

A. Post-anaesthetic or post-procedure shaking is a common occurrence after C-section. The cause is unknown, but a theory is it is an automatic stress response.

Q. Is infertility more likely after C-section? I was told I had adhesions.

A. Adhesions can cause tissue to build up inside the reproductive cavity; reproductive organs like the ovaries can be affected. It is rare.

Q. What is accreta?

A. Accreta is a severe condition where the placenta (afterbirth) can grow into the womb's deep muscle layer.

Q. My spinal anaesthetic failed: I had to go to sleep.

A. Anaesthesia carries risks, and your anaesthetist will have chosen the safest way to manage your birth anaesthetic.

Q. Why have I got a T-shaped scar on my abdomen?

A. A T-shaped scar will be for a specific medical reason. Ask your medical provider why this was necessary.

Q. Why was it so difficult to breastfeed?

A. Pain and discomfort in positioning yourself can lead to breastfeeding difficulties. Good pain management is essential, as is supportive breast positioning and attachment information.

Q. I felt guilty taking so many painkillers.

A. Pain management is the gold standard of supporting your recovery.

Q. I had comments from other people who said I 'took the easy way out' by having a C-section.

A. This type of comment is one of the reasons why the Five Guide video has been so popular. It is not the easy way out; it is major abdominal surgery. Share the video link from Chapter 2 with your sceptics.

<https://www.facebook.com/groups/728222333959968>[14] This support group highlights the many difficulties women can encounter after caesarean birth in addition to many helpful resources. Some of the questions asked were upsetting—they highlighted a lack of communication and public health education between services and patients.

What are the benefits of birth debriefing?

Very few of us can completely control our thinking. Put simply, our minds wander, and they walk a lot if you are coping with pain, tiredness, fatigue, and a crying baby. Debriefing allows you to take notice of your feelings so as not to be bottled up.

Without a birth debrief, fragmented thoughts and emotions do emerge from the kaleidoscope of our unconscious. After C-section, and particularly an emergency C-section, any unresolved emotions and feelings can lead to anxiety. They can develop into more worrying emotions, such as post-traumatic stress disorder (PTSD).[15]

The birth debrief is not about making judgments; it's about answering questions, reflecting, celebrating, exploring, and finally accepting what sensation, feeling, smell, sound, or intervention you have experienced, to allow you to move on.

Midwives and health visitors debrief women and partners in the UK. It is a nationally recognised healthcare plan, and it very often does lead to care planning that is provided for free on the National Health Service. However, in Australia, not all women will be visited at home by a maternity service nurse or midwife. Some private services and continuity of care midwifery practices can provide the type of follow-on community care afforded to UK women as part of NHS services. This is why we have joined services to celebrate the international differences, both functional and harmful, so we can bring you your virtual midwife to assist you and your recovery.

A sample guide for birth debriefing

When we are well, our mind regulates a state of engagement, and we are on automatic pilot. Following C-section and having experienced all the biological, physical, emotional, and spiritual highs and lows, it is to be expected our autopilot may 'switch off'. Birth trauma and unresolved emotional issues are very real; over 30,000 women each year are diagnosed with birth trauma issues in the UK each year.[16] Instead of the birth being a joyful experience, there could have been events that led to you now experiencing flashbacks. These events need to be discussed and resolved, just like any other traumatic life event. They will often replay again and again if not discussed, debriefed, and understood.

Use this birth debrief checklist to see If you are resolving unanswered issues that concern you. If you are not, then ask for support to get the answers you need.

Birth Debrief Checklist	Yes	No
Do you have unresolved questions about the birth?		
Did you get feedback on the care you received?		
Do you feel emotional when you reflect on the birth?		

You can access help and support through your midwifery healthcare team; just ask!

Figure 3.1 Debrief checklist

J McKnight-Cowan

Anonymous mamma's story

It wasn't until afterward that I realised I had been so focused on the actual birth—the short-term normal birth spoken so freely about—that when I reflected on my emergency section, I realised how unprepared I was. Looking at my scar, it hit home that that scar is forever my reminder to always try and be well informed in future.

Summary

Never was there a truer sentence ever spoken: 'You don't know, what you don't know.' The answers are, ironically, why this book has become a reality. Look at other women who have had a C-section: did they struggle? You can have a vantage point by using this manual to aid your self-recovery.

We have both the midwifery and child health services skills to help you and your family in your home setting. Sadly, we could only deliver this care for limited times while in employed roles. We could not possibly be there to support women twenty-four hours a day; as experts in our fields, we have looked beyond hospital care in both of our countries. And this is why this manual can provide that ongoing care, bringing it into your home by sharing with you maternity care at its best. It provides you with the practical skills and knowledge to care for yourself and know when to ask for professional help. We want to give you the courage to ask *why, when,* and *how?*— we want to empower you to recover all aspects of your wellbeing. After all, you may not have finished your family, and want to be well and confident in making informed decisions about possible future pregnancies and birth options.

References

12. NHS England » Better Births: Improving outcomes of maternity services in England – A Five Year Forward View for maternity care

13. Australian Govt Department of Health (2020). Provision of Maternity Care. Retrieved from https://www1.health.gov.au/internet/publications/publishing.nsf/Content/pacd-maternityservicesplan-toc~pacd-maternityservicesplan-chapter3#:~:text=Maternity%20care%20in%20Australia%20includes,to%20six%20weeks%20after%20birth.

14. Caesarean Section Support Australia & New Zealand—https://www.facebook.com/groups/728222333959968

15. Rowan C, Bick D, da Silva Bastos M H. Postnatal debriefing interventions to prevent maternal mental health problems after birth: exploring the gap between the evidence and UK policy and practice. Worldviews on Evidence-Based Nursing 2007; 4(2): 97–105 https://www.evidence.nhs.uk/search?q=birth+debriefing

16. Birth Trauma https://www.birthtraumaassociation.org.uk/

Chapter 4
Controlling your pain

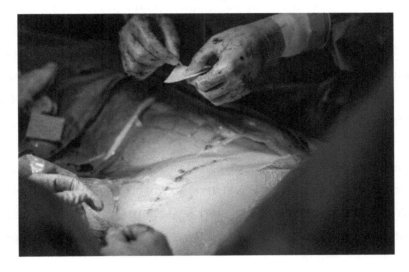

Why you should read this chapter:

- To understand your own experience of postoperative pain.
- To develop your technique in using a measurement tool to assess how bad is your pain?
- To recognise and decide on the medication, you will need to relieve your pain symptoms.
- To support you in managing pain, you can mobilise, eat, drink, and care for your baby.

Pain after C-section birth

These pretty graphic pictures tell a very different story for each woman. No matter where you live or why you have had a C-section, it hurts! Pain is a very individual feeling. No one else can see it or experience it except the person who is feeling it.

Pain management is the process of dealing with negative experiences as a result of the surgery. It is a physical and spiritual experience that requires a caring presence, courage to communicate, and compassion and respect for what a mother's beliefs and values are.

Pain has far-reaching interconnectivity with mothering, parenting, recovery, sleep, fatigue, anxiety, and emotional calmness. Problem pain connects feelings and behaviour.

Post-operative pain is an unavoidable consequence of C-section surgery. Much stretching and tugging occur during the caesarean birth process causing internal bruising and tenderness during the early days. However, the level of pain that is experienced by each woman will be unique to them.

The consequences of poorly managed pain relief will affect you physiologically and psychologically. Physiological effects will include raised heart rate and elevated blood pressure, increased respiratory effort, and sweating. An increased heart workload suggests these symptoms will, in turn, lead to psychological anxiety, anger, frustration, depression, and often crying.

Any of the factors above are unacceptable, and as a new mother post-surgery, your pain needs to be actively controlled.

If you are still in hospital and reading this manual, communicate your pain level to the nurse/midwife caring for you. Many women do not say they are in pain—they do not like to feel a burden, and they may worry it will stop them from going home. The surgery you have had involves nerves, muscle, skin, and organs. Pain is real, and it is important to understand it is part of a midwife's role to assess your postoperative pain before discharge.

The primary objective of pain assessment is to determine the severity of your pain. Not communicating this could result in the choices of pain medication being wrong for you.

Controlling your pain

Pain levels will be different at movement and rest.

Trying to slip your legs out of bed for the first time, or standing up, or reaching to comfort your baby, are all going to send you pain signals that will cause a reaction.

> Pain is whatever you say it is, existing whenever you say it does.
>
> —Janine

Pain measurement following C-section surgery needs to be simple and effective; it needs to be consistent, valid, and reliable to measure your pain.

The anaesthetist who attended you in the theatre will have assessed your pain and understood your surgery. For example, a planned, non-invasive, and routine C-section will likely not have challenged your body, mind, and spirit as much as an emergency section. It should have been more relaxed, planned, and prepared, and this can reduce some of the stressful situations an emergency will bring, including affecting your coping mechanisms.

Barriers to pain management can include emergency complications, excessive bleeding, placenta accreta, adhesions from a previous section, fetal compromise, obesity, smoking, and other medical conditions like diabetes, heart disease, low-lying placenta, and many more complications. Whether you had spinal anaesthesia or a general anaesthetic, this affects your recovery and pain sensations postoperatively.

> One C-section does not mean the same recovery for each woman, nor does it mean you will require the same pain management as the lady in the next bed to you.
>
> —Janine

Abdominal gas pains can be painful during C-section recovery and make you feel like you are about to 'lift-off'. The leading cause of gas pain is trapped air in the abdominal cavity and large intestine. After a C-section, it is typical to slow the bowel activity for several hours or days. Although this usually resolves by itself in a few days, it may be very uncomfortable. The retained gases and stool can cause the abdomen to become swollen and have painful cramps. The side effects of some pain-relieving medications following the surgery can also delay bowel activity. In some cases, hospital discharge is postponed until bowel function is restored.

Relief of gas symptoms tips

Mobilising	Get out of bed and walk as soon as possible after surgery.
Home remedies	Peppermint tea has been found to assist passing of gas. Ease cramps with hot packs to encourage passing intestinal gas as soon as possible after surgery. Gentle abdominal massage in a circular motion directed in an upside-down 'U' shape from the right-hand groin, then up and across under the ribs and down the left side can also help to mobilise the bowel into action.
Body signals	Listen carefully to your body, particularly after eating, as often the signal for a bowel movement will present around twenty minutes after eating or drinking a hot drink.
Exercises	Take some slow deep breaths and fill the lower lungs to stretch the abdominal muscles, drawing the lower back onto the bed when exhaling. The yoga posture called the 'cat stretch' can also help if you are up to it. Kneel on all fours and arch your back as you inhale and exhale, sucking in your abdominal muscles.
Positioning	Position yourself on the toilet to facilitate the bowel movement. Use a footstool to elevate your knees and a wound splint or cushion to support the incision area. Sit with a straight back while leaning slightly forward.
Medication	Stool softeners may be necessary; check with your doctor or midwife.

Figure 4.1

Remedies for wind pain (2020)

Measuring your pain—just how bad is it?

The most common pain assessment scale used in the United Kingdom with postoperative women is the numerical rating scale (NRS), which focuses on pain intensity. The tool is easy to use, reliable and takes less than a minute to complete.

Numerical Rating Scale (NRS)

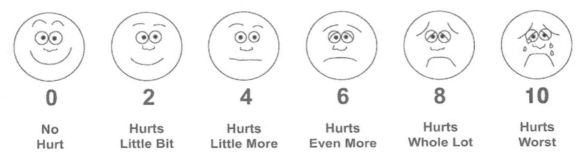

0	2	4	6	8	10
No Hurt	Hurts Little Bit	Hurts Little More	Hurts Even More	Hurts Whole Lot	Hurts Worst

https://whyy.org/segments/reassessing-the-assessment-of-pain-how-the-numeric-scale-became-so-popular-in-health-care/

How to use the numerical rating scale

Having established that you are in pain, the most appropriate way to rate your pain is to decide on what pain relief you need to manage your discomfort will become more comfortable if you follow this guide.

Key points to consider when assessing your pain

Assessing pain is multifaceted and requires careful reflection when measuring and reporting.

Key points to consider when assessing your pain	Self-assessment
How long has it been since your C-section?	Hours/Days/Weeks
Look at the scale: 0=No pain, 10=Intense pain	No pain Mild Severe
Decide on the scale where your coping mechanisms lie.	Ask yourself: *Can I cope; can I mobilise? Am I too brave?*
Decide on the scale where your pain score fits.	Take a prescribed painkiller to match your pain score.
Take pain relief according to pain scale score and safety between prescribed doses.	Remember, if the pain is persistent, ask yourself: *Am I taking the pain relief medication regularly to meet my needs?* Use your daily planner to record when you took your last medication.
How long should I use the Numerical Rating Scale?	As long as you need it.
What medication should I take?	You should take the prescribed medication you have been given.
When will I know when to stop taking medication?	Stop taking medication if you no longer need it; this could be many days for some women and up to two or three weeks for others.
Be safe self-medicating—do not take above the recommended dose.	Seek medical support and advice if your pain stays at a rating of 10 after medication.

Figure 4.2

Pain assessment

We have seen suboptimal management of pain relief amongst postoperative C-section women; this can lead to emotional and physical compromise.

Physical issues

- immobility
- constipation
- compromised feeding positions
- bladder problems
- referred pain into shoulders and back
- wind & referred shoulder tip pain
- circulatory complications
- dietary issues/low appetite.

Emotional issues

- low mood
- lack of attachment and bonding with baby
- maternal mental health anxiety
- spiritual distress
- conflict of need and ability
- negative feelings on future/past pregnancies and birth
- feeling out of control
- feeling weak or awkward/burden
- relationship issues with partner and family.

Another significant barrier to optimal pain relief management can relate to any negative perceptions and lack of knowledge of the addictive properties of opioids and analgesia side effects you may have. Please remember the anaesthetist who prescribed your medication prior to leaving hospital will be aware of any effects medication can have on breastfeeding etc.

Choice of anaesthetic

The type of anaesthetic used in a C-section will be decided in consultation with your doctor and dependent on each individual case need. A woman-centred approach ideally involves this discussion with the anaesthetist to agree on the postoperative pain management to be prescribed. If there has been a chance for a planned

C-section discussion on pain management, then the expectations of how to manage pain postoperatively can be explored and proposed. However, if the C-section is an emergency, then the opportunity can be lost. Thus, the recovery and aftermath become subjective, less controlled, and perhaps, in some cases, confusing.

As midwives, we are well trained to assess, plan, and implement pain management discussions before surgery. The fundamental difference for you in your postoperative recovery is that you also have the baby's needs to consider.

Unlike someone having a knee replacement or general surgery, women will often renounce their own needs for a safe birth.

Mothers need to function! We would all agree to that, so understanding 'normal', 'expected,' and 'acute' pain will assist your analgesia choice, combined with understanding healing pain, tissue pain, nerve pain, breast pain, uterine contraction pain, and generally feeling unwell exhaustion. Childbirth changes a woman dramatically; women go into labour often feeling physically and psychologically well, but after any type of birth will go home feeling very different.

A collaborative approach with your hospital team aims to prevent any postoperative acute pain from becoming chronic. So, initially, women may be given opioids and use a combined cocktail of medication to support their pain management needs. These will be dependent on your health, any allergies, your baby's health needs at surgery, your labour, previous medication, and a combination of general anaesthesia or spinal block anaesthesia for birth.

Anaesthetists will see you throughout your hospital stay, and they will be responsible to prescribe pain relief.

Once you are well enough, you should move around. This is encouraged usually very soon after birth once spinal anaesthesia has worn off—up to six hours after surgery is advisable, providing sensation has returned to your legs. Getting you up and moving is very important aftercare management. You will also need antithrombotic medication administered via a short needle into your abdomen. This medication is very important in helping prevent blood clots forming in the calf veins.

Pain management that is effective for home discharge is vital. It is not a sign of weakness to take the medication prescribed for your recovery.

The first twenty-four hours will be the hardest, and a combination of medication, rest, and sleep should be encouraged.

Women who are worried about the medication affecting their breast milk supply need to understand that controlling pain will lead to better outcomes in other new roles and functions as a new mother. Your choice of feeding method should be discussed with the doctor who prescribes your appropriate medication.

Medication types
Opioids
Morphine-based Class A or Schedule 8 drugs are usually prescribed in the early days.

Anti-inflammatory medications
- Paracetamol—also known as acetaminophen—is used to treat mild to moderate pain and fever
- Nefopam hydrochloride: a non-opioid and non-steroidal analgesic
- Ibuprofen.

Administration routes
- Oral
- Intravenous
- Intramuscular
- Rectal analgesia/rectal suppositories: often used after childbirth to reduce the pain experienced by women after childbirth
- Sublingual medication: taken under the tongue, this is a route of administration by which the substance is absorbed more quickly.

Non-medications

TENS machines (Transcutaneous electrical nerve stimulation)

TENS is a pain relief method involving the wearing of a small battery-operated waist-fitted device. It delivers self-controlled mild electrical currents through sticky-backed pads which fit on the skin. The electrodes fit across your back and pelvic area, and the current stimulates the natural hormonal production of an endorphin, which is the body's natural painkiller.

Acupuncture

A form of treatment that involves inserting fragile needles through a person's skin at specific points of varying depths. One hypothesis is that it works through neurohormonal pathways.

Meditation/hypnobirthing

A practice where an individual uses a technique such as mindfulness or focusing on a thought, object, or activity to train awareness and achieve a mentally apparent and emotional calmness.

Distraction techniques

A technique is simply any activity that you engage in to redirect your mind off your current emotions. Instead of putting all your energy into the upsetting feeling, you reset your attention to something else.

Cold/hot compresses

It's sometimes confusing which to use and when.

- Heat: brings more blood to the area, reduces muscle pain, should not be used in the first forty-eight hours after an injury.
- Cold: compresses ease the pain by numbing the area, reduces inflammation, reduces bleeding.

The efficacy of non-pharmacological treatments in the first few days after birth is inconclusive. Pain after C-section is real and can be intense; methods of pain relief should be thoroughly discussed and selected.

Post-operative C-section pain management is a priority as it can (and we have seen many times) lead to a long-term compromise in recovery. It can affect your quality of life to embrace new motherhood and bonding and attachment with your baby. Pain management is an individual and subjective phenomenon; each woman will react to it very differently.

The use of the prescribed medication in combination with the NRS tool will allow you to make the right choices.

You will have the control to assess your pain. Through your early days, your pain scores could be as high as ten. Over several days, you can implement your therapy to reduce and control your pain down to five or less and eventually wean yourself off any pain medication. Using your daily planners will help you to track and record your pain levels and the medication you have taken to resolve it.

Pain management

> **Gabby's story**
> The midwife's advice to me was to stay on top of the pain before I felt anything. So right on schedule of the three to four hours (or whatever the rules were), I was taking my next dose. I only did that for two to three days before I realised I didn't need that amount of pain relief. I was also advised to try to stand up and walk around (slowly and not for long) as soon as I could, and I truly believe this helped a lot with my recovery.
>
> Splinting my stitches made me feel like everything was being 'held in', I guess. I was scared of splitting my scar, but this gave me reassurance that it wouldn't happen.

Getting you up and about

Controlling your pain will allow you more time to focus on attachment and bonding with your newborn and attempt to establish feeding your baby and reflecting on the birth. Having the crib close by can ease some of the strain when attending to a baby overnight. Being able to move quickly, eat, and drink and get to the toilet, wash, and dress are normally simple tasks, however, after a C-section, some of these tasks can become huge hurdles. Use of a cushion, rolled-up towel, or dedicated splint, such as the SAC (surgical aftercare) splint,[17] to support your wound during movement can assist. Splinting the lower abdomen can give you the confidence needed to move in the early days by, in effect, providing a soft barrier against the region and holding the area stable. The SAC splint can be worn with an elasticised belt in the early days to allow you to be hands-free to carry the baby.

Post-operative pain

There are potentially many different sites you may feel pain:

- Head
- Neck
- Throat
- Shoulder tip
- Back
- Breasts
- Abdomen
- Wound sites
- Vagina
- Rectum
- Perineum
- Uterus
- Urinary catheter
- Stitches/staples
- Intravenous site
- Calf & leg

- Movement
- Clothing
- When toileting.

Rationale and remedies

Headaches

After surgery, headaches are often associated with the stress related to the procedure. If you have had a C-section and a spinal anaesthetic, ask yourself, *What type of headache is it?*

Severe headache after spinal anaesthetic

Post-dural-puncture headache is an unusual and specific kind of severe headache, which can only happen after a spinal procedure. Felt over the front and back of the head, it is worse when sitting or standing. There may be neck pain, sickness, and a dislike of bright light. Medical advice and review are necessary as a blood patch may be required. Any headache associated with drowsiness, vomiting, and confusion should be considered a medical emergency. Please then contact emergency services.

Shoulder tip pain

This is often described as a sharp stabbing pain felt in the shoulder area. Following surgery, air can become trapped in the abdominal cavity air and exert pressure on the diaphragm, which refers pain to the shoulder tip. This can be relieved with a hot pack and resolves once wind is expelled.

Throat soreness

A painful throat sometimes occurs after a general anaesthetic. Sometimes the throat can experience mild trauma when the intubation tube used to maintain your airways is inserted or removed. This can be relieved by sucking ice chips or a lozenge or taking paracetamol.

Back pain

This can be associated with pregnancy muscle changes and epidural/spinal anaesthesia procedures. Hot or cold compresses may bring some relief initially and later if persistent a massage may also help. Maintain good posture when sitting out of bed. It is also important to use a low foot stool to elevate feet.

Breastfeeding pain

The root cause of pain relating to breastfeeding can be resolved relatively quickly with the right help.

- Attachment: positioning and attachment pain can occur in the early days. It is advised not to ignore this pain as it can lead to nipple damage and further pain. Seek breastfeeding support.
- Engorgement: the breast can become overfull, resulting in tight, hard, full breasts that are painful. In the early days, milk flow will change, resulting in engorgement pain. Continue to feed and, if very engorged, express milk off the affected breast to relieve pain.
- Tongue-tie: a baby's latch can be affected by a tongue-tie that will cause difficulties in feeding and result in painful nipples. Get advice on this before your nipple is damaged.
- Blocked ducts: if you do not feed milk, glands can become engorged and result in pain. Ask for advice if you are suffering from blocked ducts. They can be very painful and lead to infection if not recognised.

Wound/abdominal pain

Incisional wound pain is very common. As the skin tissue heals at the wound site, it is painful, itchy, and sore. Abdominal pain can be associated with constipation or bowel spasms. Any sudden postoperative movement like sneezing, coughing, or even laughing can cause pain. Without adequate support and pain relief, it can lead to further complications. The SAC wound splint will help in the early postoperative days. Regular pain relief will reduce 'breakthrough' pain that causes distress. Choose a dressing you are not allergic to. Dry blood and gauze dressings, once dry, can be painful to remove. It is better to be gentle in removing wound dressings, even showering before an attempt is made to remove the dressing.

Uterus—after pains

After birth and in the subsequent days, blood loss should be bright red initially. It should not pour from you or wet a sanitary pad within an hour. Uterine pain and contracting uterine muscle are consistent with vaginal blood loss in the first few days after birth; they can often resemble menstrual cramps. They help to stem excessive bleeding by compressing blood vessels in the uterus. If there is excessive blood loss or clots, you must seek medical advice. Blood loss, also known as lochia, is natural as the lining of the uterus begins to heal. You may bleed for several days or weeks. Every woman is different. But it should not be painful, dripping blood, nor should it smell offensive. If you experience any of these symptoms, seek medical advice.

Swollen legs and ankles (oedema)

Leg swelling is often seen after birth. As the pregnancy does impede vascular return in the legs, it is common to see some leg/ankle swelling. This usually resolves in a matter of days and can be alleviated by elevating legs on a footstool and gentle foot massage.

Indwelling bladder catheters

Catheter removal will sometimes sting, especially if a spinal anaesthetic has worn off. Keeping your bladder empty is important as the pressure of a full bladder can cause pressure on your internal stitches and pain in the uterine cavity, as the bladder sits in the region of the five layers that have undergone surgery. It is rare to be discharged with a catheter due to infection risk.

Stitches, clips, or continuous suture lines

Whichever method has been used; the area will be very sore. Nerve endings in the skin are sensitive to touch and often can itch or sting as it heals. Removable sutures or clips will be painful as it is hard not to pull or tug at the sensitive skin, so be prepared and take pain relief before this procedure. Also, it is crucial if you have any surgical drains in place to have pain medication before the tubes are removed. Dressing removal will depend on the product your doctor uses. Pressure dressings are used in some facilities and need to be removed after a prescribed time to avoid pressure injury. Other dressings can be removed the next day.

Intravenous (IV) catheter

These will be removed before leaving the hospital. They have been a portal to administer medication to you, painful to have sited and can even tissue, causing hand swelling as vital IV fluid leaks into the hand/ arm. Bruising and swelling are painful, so again do not ignore the pain from these injuries, too. It might affect how you hold the baby, eat, dress, and get comfortable when at rest.

Calf /leg DVT pain

Swollen legs can be painful. Rest and elevation will reduce symptoms.

A blood clot can develop postoperatively when blood pools in the calves or thighs during bedrest or sitting for long periods. A DVT can be very serious; it is painful as the affected limb will swell. The lack of movement is often associated with inadequate pain management. Blood clots can break off and form embolisms that can lodge in vital organs, causing death. Embolisms are one of the leading causes of maternal death. Prevention is the key to management and compression stockings or thromboembolic deterrent devices (TED) stockings are prescribed to help force blood back to the heart and reduce the risk of blood pooling and clotting. While hard to put on and take off, they are lifesavers. So, getting someone to help you put those cute stocking socks on is a huge help. Another good idea is to purchase an aid such as the Caesarcare 'stocking mate' to help the tight stocking to slide easily over the ankle: the slippery fabric makes donning the socks much easier, and it can then be removed by pulling the tag through the toe hole. You will also have been prescribed blood-thinning anti-clot injections after a C-section. Using your daily planner, you can record the administration of the injections so you do not forget to administer them.

Movement

Deep breathing and coughing are essential, as are leg and ankle movements to encourage circulation and oxygenation and avoid blood clots. The ability to roll out of bed can become a huge task immediately postoperatively. Getting up and attempting to move around, even going to the bathroom, might render you feeling dizzy, unwell, and in some pain. This type of event can cause your blood pressure to go up or down.

In response to either, you will notice a feeling of being unwell. Helping yourself to help you recover will mean trying a few options, but do not stay in bed. Movement is therapy, and gentle wound splinting will support your abdomen in the early days after surgery. This is the time to start asking for help!

Be safe, feel confident, and ease yourself back into mobilising with an injury to your abdomen.

Clothing—attire/loose clothing

We all joke about the 'Bridget Jones' big knickers, but after C-section surgery, those big knickers will allow you to wear your sanitary pad more comfortably and allow your uterine scar to be free of tight obstructive clothing. Tight clothing will impede circulation and compromise your recovery time. Some women prefer firmer underwear such as bike shorts and abdominal binders; whatever your choice, be mindful of not restricting circulation and dealing with the healing process. Wounds need fresh air, light, and good hygiene.

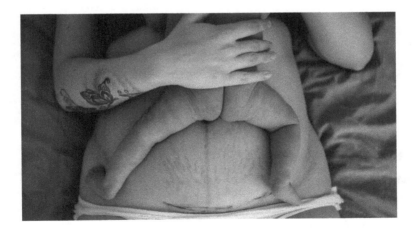

Toileting

This can be impacted by pain as you lower into position on the toilet and particularly if you experience any constipation. A cushion or splint on your lap to lean into can provide the support and confidence you need in this situation. In terms of bowel movements, a good thing to remember when keeping bowels regular is to be mindful of signals from your body after eating or having a hot drink. Your body will often begin its rumbling to eliminate waste as the new food starts to digest. Don't get constipated, as it is more painful to use your abdominal muscles to exert abdominal /rectal pushing to support eliminating stools. True constipation is not passing stools for three to five days. Time for some medicinal help if you are at that point. Keep track of your bowel habits in your daily planner otherwise it can become guesswork remembering when you last had a poo. Iron tablets can also give you constipation, that is why diet and fluids combined can help restore good toileting habits again.

15 POTENTIAL PAIN SITES FOLLOWING CAESAREAN BIRTH

1. **Headaches** may be felt as a symptom of a pre-existing condition or the epidural anaesthetic.

2. **Shoulder tip pain** may be felt like a sharp stabbing sensation in one or both shoulders..

3. **Throat soreness** may be experienced if a general anaesthetic has been used.

4. The **intravenous site** may become painful.

5. **Breast or nipple** discomfort

6. **Back pain.** the back may be tender from the spinal or epidural puncture

7. **Abdominal pain** from wind

8. **The wound area will be tender** from the surgery and possible bruising.

9. **Wound infection** or a **surgical wound breakdown.**

10. **Shock, grief, emotional trauma and pain.**

11. **Spiritual distress** especially after a traumatic emergency c-section.

12. The **urinary catheter** into the bladder may cause discomfort.

13. **Calves** may become hot and swollen.

14. **Ankles** may be tight and uncomfortable.

15. **Mental health issues**, postnatal anxiety & depression

Figure 4.3 Potential Pain Sites
L Rastas & J McKnight-Cowan.

Managing Pain at Home

When at home, remember any medication you have is not to stock up your medicine cabinet; it is there for you. Use your daily planner to record your times when taking pain relief so you can take doses on time and keep ahead of the pain to avoid unnecessary peaks.

Sitting in a chair to eat and drink, get up, sit up, and let your food be absorbed and digested properly. Trying to eat and drink when in so much pain will result in you likely refusing food. Balanced nutrition and vitamins are vital to your healing and your recovery.

When bathing babies, be mindful of the height of the bath—not too high or low to avoid strain. Get your partner to fill and empty the bathtub.

Bathing: yes, you can have a moderately warm bath a few days after surgery. It is good to remove the operative dressing within three days, as long as it is safe to do so. First check with your medical team. There are surgical dressings available, called PICO,[18] a negative-pressure wound therapy dressing for closed surgical incision wounds. This can stay on for seven days. Most are waterproof; however, if yours is not, then you can still shower after birth. The best advice is to keep the wound clean and dry. Pat dry with a wound towel—not used anywhere else but to pat dry your scar. Avoid beauty products in the bath or topical products onto the injury. If the wound is weeping a little bit, a sterile dressing must be applied, not a sanitary pad, as they have unsterile absorbent gels in them, which is not conducive for wound healing.

Why does it hurt when I move?

Any movement involving your core muscles and five layers of abdominal healing will exert some strain on your stitches. To help keep the discomfort to a minimum, it is good practice to support the wound with a splinting device, cushion, or rolled-up towel. This is especially helpful for sudden movements such as coughing, sneezing, and laughing. Sudden movements cause the pressure in the abdominal cavity to increase during the event, which can exert stress, known as mechanical stress, on the internal stitches, and in some cases, cause the wound to open. It is good practice to have your support device nearby at all times and ideally attached by a belt for easy access. It will usually only be needed for the first few weeks until the healing process strengthens the wound, and it becomes less vulnerable.

Figure 4.4 The SAC (surgical after care) wound splint

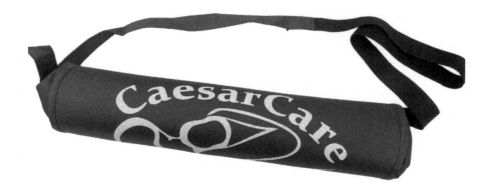

How does a wound splint work?

The splint, when placed gently across the stitches and held firmly against the area, helps to counter or reduce the forward thrust of the muscles during movement, particularly sudden changes. Being able to support the wound like this provides the confidence needed to stay mobile.

You can quite simply splint your wound with a rolled-up towel, cushion, or another dedicated device such as Caesarcare's SAC splint.

Figure 4.5 Towel splint

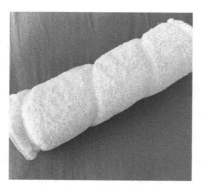

The SAC splint is particularly useful when moving from sitting to a standing position and for support while walking. You may find it helpful when using the toilet also to sit with the splint, towel, or cushion on your lap and lean into it as you pass a stool.

Keep your splinting device close to you while in bed in case of any sudden movement such as coughing, sneezing, or laughing, so you have easy access to support your wound. Some SAC splints have elasticised belts attached to provide a wearable feature for ready access and allow you to be hands-free to carry your baby. The comfort and confidence that comes with splinting your wound are well worth considering.

Kirsty's story

My partner and both set of grandparents were amazing, offering help to wash, cook, walk the dog, and simply support me in my recovery, never once taking my baby away from me.

Summary

In summary, pain is only yours to feel and yours to own and act upon accordingly. More pain equals less mobility and less enjoyment of the birth experience. Do not suffer in silence; be active and take charge of your day and your recovery by making pain a number one priority to manage. C-section is not an easy way out; it is major abdominal surgery, and the process is the result of five abdominal layers surgically opened to deliver your baby.

Skin, fat, muscle, peritoneal layer, and then uterus are all opened to deliver your baby. Those five layers will take up to six weeks to heal, repair, and recover.

Only when the initial healing process has taken place will you be able to consider then moving onto other supportive methods to enhance your recovery.

Top Tip

Pain relief will be prescribed; it is advised you make an informed decision on measuring your pain levels by using the numerical rating scale (NRS), score your initial pain, and include your chosen method of pain relief to eliminate any unnecessary suffering. Using the NRS will allow you to make the right choices to improve your mobility and general wellbeing.

Well-managed pain will enable you to move about more freely and comfortably so you enjoy caring for and bonding with your baby.

References

17. SAC splint https://www.caesarcare.com/blog?tag=wound+breakdown

18. PICO Wound dressing: retrieved from https://www.nice.org.uk/guidance/MTG43

Chapter 5
Leaving hospital and adjusting to home

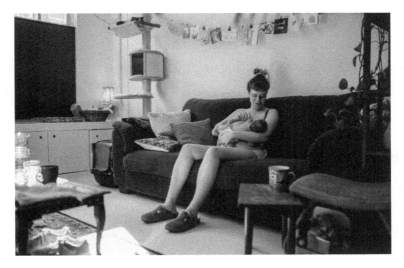

Why you should read this chapter:

- To explore how to be a new mum with a baby, a home, and trying to recover from C- section surgery.
- To learn how to ask for help, share with your support network what is the most valuable thing you will benefit from in your early days and weeks of your recovery.
- To help you understand your reaction and emotions, avoiding the pitfalls of inability vs. ability, this chapter should help you gain independence.
- To help look at the artistry of homecoming vs. the social science of expectation and preparation, with positive virtual midwifery tips to enhance your homecoming experience.

You are probably asking *what*, *why*, and *how*, which are all key to avoiding disappointment in yourself and others. This whirlwind of planning, preparation, excitement, joy can be mixed with sadness, pain, disappointment, guilt, shame, and fear. The reality of who you now are and what your new role is can suddenly be upon you, and for first-time mothers especially, it can be quite a bombshell! During our observations and experiences as hospital and community midwives, we have both seen the good days, the bad, the joy, the sadness, the smiles, and the tears.

It is here we wanted to share with you our experiences and help answer the *what*, *why*, and *how-to-fix-it* list for transitioning to coming home.

> Number one piece of advice: rest, and enjoy your baby!
>
> —Anonymous mamma

Some key considerations and suggestions for coming home with baby

The following list of topics has been inspired by both our professional and personal experience, and we offer them to help you better prepare for coming home with your baby or babies.

Is the home ready?

A messy home will encourage you not to function well. If you are usually a tidy homemaker, then preparation is the key. Use the support network around you: your partner, your parents, and your friends to help you recover and take on some domestic household chores for you. Being too proud to ask can result in personal conflict. Don't be afraid to reach out for help; remember the Five Guide lesson—you have every right to ask for help.

Do we have enough food at home?

Without the right nutritious food postoperatively, you will challenge your recovery to heal. Stock the freezer up with nourishing everyday food that only requires reheating in the first weeks after birth.

Accept offers to cook for you and your family by your support network. Be sure to alert them to any food intolerances. We encourage you to use your daily planner to track your meals, as the hours run into a blur as you care for your baby day and night it is easy to lose track of mealtimes.

Do I have enough help at home?

You will need a full six weeks to recover from your operation. Some women find it helpful to engage a postpartum doula in the first few weeks to help with all chores around the baby and home but there is a charge for these services. If the world around you seems to fall apart, you may feel the same way too. Your priority is to heal from your surgery and learn to be the mother you hoped to be. Other tasks can get in the way; how you deal with them is vital. Accepting help for yourself, your family, and your home will allow you to embrace time with your new baby and explore attachment, bonding, and perhaps focus on breastfeeding or your recovery more. There are no tired and fatigued hero mothers. Family and friends can be your best source of help if you can let them know how they can best help and support you during your recovery time. People are willing to help, but often it's hard to think on the spot, so keeping a list or whiteboard of tasks can be an effective way to delegate without the stress of on-the-spot thinking.

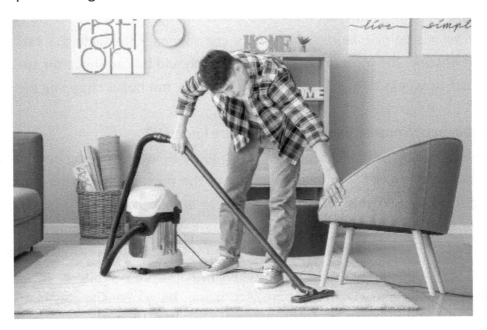

Who will do the laundry?

There will be more laundry than ever. Baby clothes and sheets add to the load of washing your family already created. Soiled bed linen from uterine bleeding, extra bathing towels, and all the baby muslins, nappies, and day clothes will build up every day. But, after surgery, these roles need to be delegated for a while. A supportive network of willing visitors can come in handy for washing laundry, pegging it out, and ironing it. It makes visitors to your home feel wanted and useful. Everyone wants to help—even with the dirty stuff—so let them. You are not fit enough to do it yet.

A top tip is to purchase or make a chores board, then as each visitor comes to see you and new baby, they can choose a chore to help you, like bed changing, duvet change, laundry folding/ironing, pop to the grocers for you etc.

Who will do the grocery shopping?

Online grocery shopping is great after a baby is born. In the comfort of your own home, you and your family can order your grocery items. It's best to avoid getting out to the stores after surgery, especially as you are not safe to drive in the first few weeks. The decision to operate a car is supported by asking yourself, *Could I easily do an emergency stop or take the impact of a car accident?* Delegate this task to your support network. The most important thing you should be carrying after surgery and for the first six weeks is the weight of your new baby, not heavy shopping bags.

Will all the baby/mother equipment be where I need it?

When you get home, the last thing you need to be doing is opening new packets of baby clothes to launder. Timely preparation of the nursery and clothing is advised. If not, get help to do this. Organising a system around caring for a baby can help eliminate unnecessary stress. A support network of friends and family feel part of the baby's world if they are allowed to help you set up the nursery and support your needs to make coming home more natural for you. Include your items: sanitary pads, big knickers, loose clothing, breast pads, etc. If your baby needs to stay in hospital or is in the neonatal unit, we strongly advise you to ask for help. Long days and tiring nights are spent by many a mother and family in neonatal units, desperate to be with their baby but, in some cases, also have other children to care for. Make this transition period as easy for yourself as you can. Wouldn't it be great to come home from the hospital to a cooked meal, the house tidy, and the laundry all done?

Asking for help is a sign of recovery and positive parenting.

What about other family members?

Siblings, depending on their age, can increase the workload and stress for their poor mum. Small children will have little or no understanding of what being gentle, quiet, or less excited should mean. Small siblings can react quite negatively toward a new baby and not understand why Mummy cannot roll around the floor at the moment. Family members would benefit from seeing the Five Guide video[19] to support their knowledge of what has happened to you, and in turn, help your recovery more. Do communicate how and why you need their help. With small children, sleep when they do, eat with them, and try to maintain their routines. Smaller siblings do benefit from gender play roles when a new baby arrives, so getting a doll and toy feeding bottle is always a good role-model play activity.

> **Anonymous twin mamma**
>
> My babies—twin girl and boy—were delivered at 30 weeks. I couldn't drive for six weeks. That was probably the hardest thing to accept. I needed to be ferried to and from the NICU which meant I needed to be grateful and calm. I rarely was, and none of my lovely drivers—friends, family, and daddy—ever complained to me.

Will I be able to drive?

Ideally, not in the first few weeks. Ask yourself:

- Can I move freely?
- Could I do an emergency stop?
- Will my insurance company cover me in the event of an accident?

- Am I in pain?
- Am I feeling faint?
- Am I feeling well enough?

It is safer to wait six weeks to allow your abdominal muscles to heal. Five layers of the abdominal cavity are injured; it takes six weeks for it to heal surgically. Your postpartum period is six weeks long for a reason. Rely on a supportive network as much as you can in this period of your recovery.

How long will it take to recover?

It will take 5–6 weeks for the wound to heal providing there are no surgical wound complications such as infection or burst stitches.

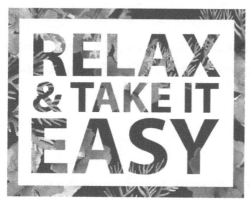

Remember five layers are healing:
1. Skin
2. Fat layer
3. Muscle layer
4. Peritoneal sack
5. Uterus/womb.

Each layer should heal independently of the other, but sometimes adhesions form.

Adhesions form when internal layers heal inclusively and cause the tissue to adhere to each layer to one another or an organ like the bladder or bowel. Recovery also depends on health, rest, nutrition, blood loss at birth, wound care, and pain management. In theory, you should feel improvement in your physical healing by week five to six. Long-term recovery will take up to a year. Lie down each afternoon and take a power nap. If you do this, you allow your stomach anatomy to rest, recover, and heal. Keep your bowels empty, don't strain, and avoid constipation. Keep your bladder empty; this will avoid pressure in your uterine cavity.

Take your prescribed medication.

Take iron tablets to support haemoglobin (red blood cell) repair and growth.

Eat well, and drink plenty of fluids like water but avoid tea and coffee as they contain tannins, which inhibit the absorption of iron from your diet or iron tablet medication. Multivitamins support tissue repair. Remember, every woman is different. If you allow yourself to know your body and its limits, listen to your body, read the signs of fatigue, pain, and injury. Then you will be allowing the healing process to develop, and recovery will be supported. Build up walking daily: walking helps prevent blood clots and constipation. Walk every day, building up distance slowly every day. Use your daily planner to keep track of medication, diet, and all the tasks you need to perform in your recovery journey. Tiredness and fatigue will blur the times and schedules you normally are on top of.

What if I can't reach across to the baby easily?

Having the baby near you is recommended. A low crib can be difficult to reach in the early days, so help and support are vital. We use our abdominal muscles for all core movements: in and out, up and down, across and above. Every way you used to move before birth is typically temporarily changed. Your body will send out signals of pain, and you can lack strength and ability in most routine tasks. However, this is short-term. You are advised to read the section on pain management. The key to more effortless mobility is pain management and a focus on your complete recovery. Self-care in terms of pain, wound management, blood loss, diet, sleep, and rest are important considerations. Use a rolled-up towel or the SAC splint to support your abdominal movements.[20]

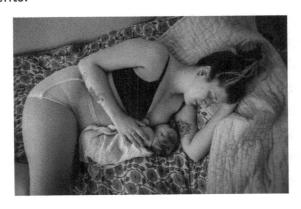

A bedside, adjustable height crib can be beneficial, but you can also raise a lower crib on a firm surface to make reaching the baby at night easier.

Safe sleeping position for baby

How a baby lies to sleep is now a widely recognised safety priority. Check out safe sleep positions and cot safety advice online.[21]

- Baby should be on its back, never on its tummy
- The baby should be put into a separate crib and placed feet to the bottom
- Baby should ideally sleep in the same room as parents for 6–12 months
- Use a firm, flat waterproof mattress, with no gaps around the edges
- No bumpers or toys in the cot to avoid the risk of suffocation
- Never sleep in an armchair or bed with your baby
- Baby should not be wearing a hat or have covers over its head
- Baby shouldn't be propped upright or over onto its side with blankets or padding
- Room temperature ideally between 16–20°C
- Keep baby in a smoke-free zone.

Sharing a sleep surface with the baby is not advised by health authorities owing to the risk of fatal sleep accidents such as sudden unexpected death in infancy (SUDI) or sudden infant death syndrome (SIDS).[22] This topic can be explored further by accessing these valuable resources at <https://www.unicef.org.uk/babyfriendly/news-and-research/baby-friendly-research/infant-health-research/infant-health-research-bed-sharing-infant-sleep-and-sids/>.

What if I can't hold the baby easily?

Your abdominal muscles are core to any movement. Holding the baby and experiencing associated abdominal scar pain? Then try reading Chapter 4; there are lots of top tips to help you. The problem will affect how you control your movements. Holding the baby close to you will be difficult initially. You may have had intravenous needles in your hands or arms, and they are likely to be swollen, sore, and bruised. Your energy level, skills, and techniques to hold your baby will grow as you nurture your complete recovery. Try different positions:

- Lie down on your side to feed or hold the baby.
- Sit supported with pillows, rest the baby on your lap.
- Try a baby sling to support your back and bring the baby closer to you.
- The 'rugby ball' hold is also a great tip, rather than across the body. The baby is tucked under your arm and supported with a pillow underneath.

Be creative, be positive, and hold your baby; attach and bond with your little miracle.

What if I am in pain?
The scale of discomfort caused by post-C-section surgery is a very individual thing.

No one can see it, and only you can feel it. Being aware of how you can manage this is the key. Please go to Chapter 4 to learn how to understand, manage, and prevent your pain engulfing your early days of motherhood. Pain is inevitable following this surgery: suffering is not. Yours to own and prevent. Nerves, skin, muscle, fat layer, and uterus have been under assault to birth you to your baby. They will react by sending out all the symptoms of pain in your skin, body, arms, legs, feet, shoulders, back, head, etc.

Pain has far-reaching interconnectivity with mothering, parenting, recovery, sleep, fatigue, anxiety, and emotional calmness. Pain impacts feelings and behaviour.

Use the numerical rating scale (NRS) to measure your pain and treat it with medication accordingly.[23] Revisit the management of your pain regularly.

Anxiety can cause pain to feel worse, so regularly check yourself for root causes of stress and anxiety and work to reduce them. Daily planner tracking will keep you on time with your medication needs.

I need iron tablets, but I am constipated
You may have a low blood haemoglobin level, causing anaemia from blood loss. It is essential that is corrected with supplements; however, a side effect of the iron supplement may be constipation. Drink at least one–two litres of water daily and eat

foods with high fibre content to help soften the stools; a stool softener may also be necessary. Start your day with a high-roughage cereal and a piece of fruit, as this has good bulky fibre for the bowel. Avoid juices as they are high in sugar, and a hot toasty slice of wholemeal bread is much healthier than white bread. Favour brown carbs like brown pasta and rice as the energy from these foods is longer lasting and adds fibre to your bowel. Iron supplements are important; you must take the prescribed course and regulate any side effects with diet and fluids

Why do I need iron tablets?

You may be prescribed iron supplements and will need to take the course prescribed. Iron supplements are minerals that are vital to your health and blood quality to recover. The reason you need them is most likely to be blood loss during birth. For optimal absorption of iron, it is recommended to take vitamin C or juices rich in vitamin C. Iron supplements can be liquid form or tablet form, and some foods have useful iron minerals in them. Iron supplements restore the normal function of red blood cells in your recovery. Red blood cells are required to heal, make breast milk, and restore blood volume to a healthy level. Symptoms of anaemia include fatigue, tiredness, shortness of breath, headaches, poor appetite, and pale colour. Iron is needed to support skin tissue healing.

What if I feel unwell?

Feeling very unwell is a symptom where your body will send you specific signals. Do not ignore them. High temperatures, shivers, pain, offensive wound odour, wound oozing, headaches, nausea, whatever the symptom, your body is trying to tell you something; it is important to listen to it and consult a health professional.

Postoperative complications can occur. This section is designed to help you focus and be alert to your signs and symptoms. When you are no longer able to control them, or they have been with you for more than a few hours, seek advice from your healthcare professional to ensure timely identification and treatment of complications.

Remember, there is no problem too small to discuss; prevention is better than cure. No one can help if no one knows.

What if I am feeling stressed?

Stress and fatigue are common feelings after surgical birth and can be reactions to mental or emotional pressure. However, if you had a history of stress before the baby arrived, then your coping mechanisms may be less effective. Stress shows itself in many forms: crying, fatigue, temper, headaches, and, in some cases, losing control.

Stress happens when the body feels under pressure, so it is important to find a coping mechanism that is safe for you and your baby. Taking a relaxing bath and getting your support network to know you are feeling stressed is essential. The body reacts to stress with a chemical reaction releasing the hormone cortisol which is also known as the 'raging' hormone.

Stress is your body's way to get you to sense danger, so listen to your body.

It may be difficult for you to pin down exactly why you are stressed. It doesn't matter. Your reaction to the feeling does. Share your feeling with your family, get help, rest, and seek professional help if it doesn't go away. Aromatherapy, massage, yoga, acupuncture, and music therapy can also provide relief from stress and discomfort.[24]

What if I feel like a failure?

Women can experience feelings of failure, guilt, and shame about their birth outcome being different from their hopes. This is common for women who have had an emergency C-section. You may have had a different birth all planned out and never envisaged what has happened to you. Why would you? One in four women experience a C-section: it is not a failure to have tried and not given birth naturally. Think back and reflect on your birth debrief in Chapter 3. There is a reason you did not or could not have your baby vaginally; seek answers to help understand your feelings. Having a baby was never an experiment to fail or pass. A C-section was your baby's safe passage into this world. Depending on your health and obstetric history, you may be able to try for vaginal birth in future pregnancies. For some women, this is their journey into motherhood. We know just what a warrior you are and what your body has been through to deliver you of your baby.

But you alone need to process this, and you need to know why, what, and how things happened to you. A birth debrief is a right; you really need to know what happened to you and why to support your recovery. We advise you not to carry this emotional burden—revisit Chapter 3 and take a look at the debrief check list. If you answer 'yes' to the questions, plan to seek help from your maternity healthcare team to discuss and resolve.

What if I do not feel bonded with the baby?

Bonding and *attachment* are the terms used to explore the emotional connection formed between mother and baby. Neither go hand in hand, and often after a traumatic and stressful birth, the experience of bonding can be interrupted. Bonding can be supported after a C-section with actions like skin-to-skin contact, where the newborn baby is put directly onto a mother's chest, almost naked—nappy advised!

Bonding is not the same as an attachment: parents *bond* with their children, baby *attaches* to their mother and father by smell, touch, sensory, breastfeeding, and skin-to-skin contact. Try this in your quiet times with a baby that is well-fed, warm, and just look and gaze at the miracle you have delivered. Over the hours and days after a C-section birth, this can take a little longer to experience. Hang in there; it will develop, and then you will never look back.

I can't remember what happened to me

The human brain can suppress trauma, lessen it, or enhance it. The brain will code it and place it into our unconscious memory.

The birth debrief, if done with your birth partner, will help you to reflect on this experience. It will boost performance in your brain to decide what is essential information for you to process and what is not. Partners often shoulder and protect women from what happened in emergencies. It is crucial to consider the birth debrief if needed for a partner too. Remember, what they saw you go through may have made them feel helpless and worried and left them feeling traumatised. Partners may benefit from counselling also.

Who will come to see me from the medical team?

Health professionals home visiting will depend on where you live and the offer of community care. A home visit is a luxury in some countries. Women in the UK get up to five postnatal visits from health professionals after birth. Whoever comes to see you, make it work in your favour. Ask your questions and know what is required and why. The baby will also need tests and reviews. Maternity support teams include doctors, nurses, midwives, doulas, maternity support workers, district nurses. Some of their visits will be scheduled and some unannounced, so be prepared to be examined, have your wound checked, and your baby reviewed. In Australia, home visits are not as common—mothers take their baby to a maternal and child health centre for assessment and support. Show and tell them about anything that concerns you.

Why do I need to take the abdominal injections?

Thromboglobulin is the correct name for the postoperative injection therapy women have after abdominal surgery.

You need this to prevent blood clots. The injections are an anticoagulant or blood thinner and are administered as prescribed by a doctor. Women may be sent home with the injections and a safety needle dispenser. Along with your theatre stockings, the injections will help reduce your likelihood of a severe blood clot disorder. Keep mobile, get up and dressed, washed and fed, but rest for power naps during the day.

Why have I got to wear special stockings?

TED stockings—or anti-embolism stockings—are clinically-proven compression socks to wear. Most come up to the knee and are difficult to put on, but there is a specific sock slipper to help you pop them on and off. The stockings help prevent blood clots from forming while you are less mobile. They also help reduce swollen ankles as you recover. A condition called deep vein thrombosis (DVT) is a severe complication requiring urgent medical care. You must adhere to wearing them until told otherwise. They guard against a severe postoperative complication. Early postoperative antithrombotic needles are also given to help prevent this condition arising. Keep track of this using your daily planner to record that you have had the injection administered.

Why do I need to get out of bed?

Being or becoming bedridden leads to many postoperative complications; however, it is relatively healthy after your C-section to enjoy an afternoon nap. If you lie down and rest when your baby is sleeping, you will be restoring valuable, healthy body nutrients. You should not stay in bed unnecessarily. In the past, women took to their beds after having a baby; this resulted in blood clots forming. Gentle mobilisation and deep breathing are beneficial for your recovery; the more you move, the less stiffness you will feel.

Why is back care important?

It's essential to look after your back after having a baby. Pregnancy can make your ligaments and muscles weaker. Don't lift anything heavier than your baby for the first six weeks.

These are some things you can do to help protect your back:

- Avoid bending over low tables/beds. Try having work surfaces at belly-button height.
- When you have to lift something, draw in your pelvic floor muscles and your tummy muscles. Don't hold your breath. If you are sitting on the floor with a baby, try leaning your back against something for support and don't hunch.

Why avoid too much tea and coffee?

Tannins are a type of plant compound naturally found in foods and drinks like tea, coffee, and chocolate. They inhibit the absorption of iron. So, if you are on iron supplements for low haemoglobin, then it's wise to try to avoid drinking too much.

Try to drink plenty of fluids to enhance your recovery: water and juices. Avoid gassy drinks as they will give you wind and may give rise to abdominal wind and pain.

Why should I go for an afternoon lie-down?

The value of an afternoon nap after a C-section can't be overstated. Healthy recovery postoperatively isn't just for babies. Mothers' coping mechanisms and wound recovery will improve with a regular afternoon nap. An afternoon nap is one of the joys of new motherhood. Get up feeling refreshed and ready for the continued care you give to you and your baby. Napping is not being lazy—it is vital to recovery. Indulge and enjoy. We always advise a power nap daily until you feel you do not need it anymore. Sleep is energy, and energy helps you to cope and recover. Sleep is also important for the production of the hormone prolactin and building up milk supply if you are breastfeeding your baby.

When should I do pelvic floor exercises?

In our experience, it is a myth that pelvic floor exercises are not necessary unless you have a vaginal birth; strength needs to be regained after all the weight and stretching that has taken place. Strengthening your pelvic floor muscles can reduce the likelihood of urinary incontinence. It can also enhance vaginal muscle strength and help support a healthy sex life. Even with a C-section birth, pelvic floor muscle exercises are essential. You may also have tried to deliver vaginally and have more wounds to heal, especially after labouring, dilation, failed induction, and subsequent attempts to vacuum-extract or forceps-deliver the baby. An episiotomy will also weaken the vaginal wall in varying degrees.

Pelvic floor muscles can be felt if you try stopping the flow of urine at peeing. Hold for a few seconds, then release. Feel the tightening of the muscles. Rectal muscles also need to be strengthened and included in exercises. Identifying which is a skill, initially—women we have cared for we asked to imagine they need the toilet and to stop wetting or soiling themselves. Then squeeze either your vagina or your rectum tightly, holding that for at least ten seconds. This is a pelvic floor exercise; it tightens up the affected muscles in the lower pelvis. Tightening these muscles for five to ten seconds each day at each toilet visit will develop into a pelvic workout.[25]

How do I get out of bed safely?

Just can't make it out of bed? Are you tired, in pain, have weak muscles, or just not feeling up to it? Whatever the reason, you need help to get started. Painful abdominal muscle actions are usually the cause. Make sure you have measured your pain and taken pain relief before you try. Are stitches sore or pulling? Then consider using a rolled-up towel or the Caesarcare splint to support your tummy (see Chapter 4, 'How does a wound splint work?'). If your bed is lower and more challenging to get yourself up, try more pillows, and get a second person to help you.

Rolling onto your side, pushing yourself up with your lower elbow while pushing the head of the bed with your upper arm is better than trying to bend in the middle. Ease your feet over the bedside first and then compose yourself before trying to stand. Remember, you might feel a little faint at first, so be safe and take your time!

Spiritual self-care

Childbirth affects all dimensions of the human condition. The human spirit may have been troubled by the birth and often needs to be listened to, nurtured, energised, and celebrated after the birth of a baby. When we do not achieve the birth we hoped for due to emergency surgery or delayed intensive care recovery, we can experience spiritual distress. Taking time to nurture your spirit and heal and recover becomes as essential as food. Try scheduling time for whatever it is that feeds your spirit, for example, being in nature, spiritual reading, meditation, prayer, yoga, song, or so on— whatever helps you transcend moments in time to foster a sense of healing, awe, love, hope, and centring on meaning and purpose in this new gift of life. This is where recording your emotions and feelings in your journal will help you to process your behaviour. Reflection can be a powerful gift, and as you begin to feel stronger, you can see the journey you are taking into recovery.

What about any tummy overhang, pouch, or C-section shelf and diastasis?

These take time and targeted exercise to resolve, which is difficult when wound pain restricts activity. There will be some shelf or pouch of abdominal swelling long after surgery; a baby stretched it to grow and be born. Now your body will heal and eventually you can focus on regaining your pre-baby weight and shape.

After six weeks, you can begin a gentle exercise. Discuss this with a physiotherapist who can help you with practical activities or perhaps some online classes.[26] Don't be too hasty, and remember this scar is a badge of honour for your C-section birth—wear it with pride.

Please pace yourself and do not overdo it—there are five layers all competing to heal, and you want them to heal independent of another, so recover slowly.

Figure 5.1 C-section overhang

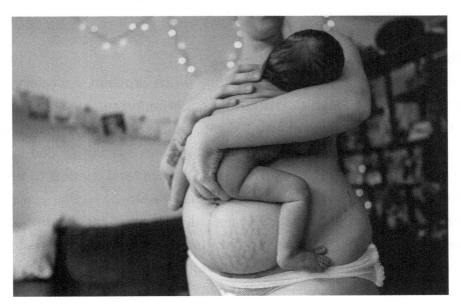

What is the best way to pick things up from the floor?

You will find it challenging to use your core abdominal muscles to bend. In the first weeks, your stomach muscles will be bruised and sore. The most comfortable action is to ask someone else to help you first. Do not overstretch; it can do internal damage, and then you will regret not asking. Squatting is the preferred position, and using an 'easy reacher' or 'grabber stick' is a helpful tool for picking things off the floor.

How can I carry the baby?

How to lift and carry your baby from place to place will require the use of arm strength and abdominal muscles. Safety and care are needed; practice will make perfect. There are a few things to remember when you are carrying a baby: support their head and have a firm safe hold on them so they do not wriggle free.

In the first few hours and days, as your confidence grows, you may experience some pain when performing this task. Try to always be at the baby's level: not bending down or across will make lifting babies easier. Initially, it will drag on the wound to be carrying anything more substantial than the baby. Enjoy skin-to-skin time together after a C-section. Certain positions are more comfortable for you to learn to hold your baby. The classic hold across your stomach may not initially be the most comfortable. So, try looking at these pictures to choose a hold that best suits you.

What about constipation?

Many women say that constipation was their worst problem, especially as a side effect of some pain relief medication. Positioning is important; ideally, with feet on a low stool so your knees can be elevated slightly above hip level. Lean forward when you sit on the toilet and rest your elbows on your knees. Placing a rolled-up towel or splint on your lap to lean into can help provide support and comfort to the wound. Relax your belly and keep your back straight. Breathe slowly so that you don't hold your breath. If you have to push hard to get the poo out, it can weaken your pelvic floor muscle in the long term. Drink lots of water and eat fruit and veggies to keep the poo soft and smooth to push out. If constipation persists, some laxative medication may be necessary.

When should I seek medical help?

If you experience any of the listed issues within the first six months after the birth of your baby, seek medical advice:

- Back, neck, tailbone, or wrist pain.
- Painful scar tissue.
- Pain during sexual intercourse.
- Weak or separated stomach muscles.
- Bladder or bowel problems.
- Emotional health issues.
- Breast pain/lumpiness.
- Pelvic floor weakness or vaginal 'heaviness'.

Postpartum headaches

These can occur anytime in the first six weeks after birth. Sometimes headaches can occur as an after-effect of the spinal or epidural anaesthetic and can persist even when lying down. This type of headache is caused by a subdural haematoma, so if the headache hasn't improved after twenty-four hours, your doctor must be informed. Your doctor may decide to administer a blood patch to remedy the problem. This is done by injecting a small amount of your blood into the epidural or spinal area, which will then restore normal pressure in the spinal fluid and relieve the headache. Early diagnosis is important so be sure to report any headaches.

Why are my feet and legs swollen after birth?

Postpartum swollen leg (oedema) is common and should naturally disappear with rest and leg elevation. After birth, any postpartum swelling that is also hot, in just one leg, or is painful could be symptomatic of a blood clot or DVT (deep vein thrombosis).

It is advisable to wear your antithrombotic socks as advised and, if concerned, seek medical advice.[27]

What about visitors after the baby is born?

Managing your visitors after your baby is born via C-section is essential. It's understandable that you'll be excited to introduce your beautiful baby to family and friends as soon as possible, but remember your baby needs time alone to get to know you and your partner's voices, touch, and scent. We have seen many postnatal rooms jam-packed with excited family and friends all wanting to cuddle the baby within hours of birth. Not only can this be exhausting for the mother, but it can also be confusing for the baby being passed between different people. If you can wait twenty-four hours, it would be better. Once home, it's a good idea to develop a schedule for visitors and use them as a support network to help you, not a time for you making tea at the expense of tiredness and fatigue. A valuable resource to support you: <https://www.babylist.com/hello-baby/how-to-manage-visitors-after-baby-comes>.

What causes postoperative shaking?

The involuntary muscular activity associated with post-anaesthetic shaking or shivering can be quite alarming. It is the body reacting to the surgery, fluid loss, and medication you will have received. It is common, and the cause is associated with a drop in core body temperature. It is good practice to receive warmed intravenous fluids during surgery to avoid this happening. It can leave you with quite a bad memory; this is best discussed in a birth debrief (please review Chapter 3).

Accepting help

Visitors can be a great source of help in those early recovery days, so delegate; your visitors will feel they are helpful if you let them help you. Remember, in many cultures, the birthing mother is supported by women in the village or live-in family members, and help is inbuilt. You have every reason to welcome offers of help.

Leave the housework, relax, and embrace just how your body is communicating to you; it's healing. Becoming in tune with your body will allow you to respond to pain, infection, and maternal mental health anxieties.

Your body and your recovery need you to be an active participant; only then will you invest in your recovery needs and enjoy coming home.

Suggestions for practical help and support your friends, family, or postnatal doula may help with:

Regular tasks

- dishes
- meal preparation
- washing and ironing
- grocery shopping
- cleaning.

Baby-related tasks

- nappy changing
- bathing baby
- folding baby clothes
- soothing the baby between feeds
- minding baby to allow afternoon nap.

Mother-related tasks

- keep food and fluids a priority
- help limit visitor stay times
- talk about the birth experience
- arrange for the mother to speak to a professional if needed
- offer to help with personal shopping
- offer to mind baby whilst mother takes time out.

Raylene's story

The hardest part for me was relying on others for help. I have always been an independent person, and now I am a single mother having to rely on others for the little things like driving to the shops, lifting, and hanging washing on the line, etc. I guess I underestimated that a C-section is major surgery, and taking it easy for the recovery period is important and a must. I just had to slow down and convince myself that it's okay if things don't get done today, and once I got my head around that, I really embraced motherhood and the special bonding time I was having with my daughter. I also realised that I wasn't being a burden, and my mum was completely happy to help out.

When I was still in hospital and was sipping on a cup of tea and it went down the wrong way and I coughed, it felt like my insides were ripping. From then on, the splint was right beside me for any coughing, laughing, etc., episodes. The SAC splint definitely helped!

Summary

In our experience, coming home after a C-section can cause a mixed bag of emotions: fear, anxiety, love, doubt, and excitement. You will possibly experience them all in varying degrees at some stage, both negative and positive.

You have been through an incredibly physical event, and you and your recovery are as paramount as all the joys and celebrations of bringing home your new baby.

But if you have had to leave your baby behind in a neonatal unit (NNU), then you may want to reflect on this time at home as an opportunity to regain all your strength for the subsequent hospital visits and parenting journey ahead.

Women discharged home before their baby can experience many physical and emotional hurdles. The main focus is recovery: if you are to be your baby's strength, you are going to need all of yours.

Expectations to express breast milk when there are no baby cues, like crying and feeding nipple-to-nipple, does add to the difficulties you may experience in your recovery.

Sleep, rest, and recovery should be essential; sitting for long hours in the NNU is not suitable for your physical recovery. Pace your visits against sleep, good food, and pain medication needs. Use the recovery manual just the same: record your daily journal. This is as important as getting the wellbeing handover on your baby from the NNU team.

Once home, all the joys and tribulations will unfold as family life begins. Hopefully, your partner will be on paternity leave, and their support is vital to aid your recovery. Coming home is just the beginning of a new role. A new baby takes time to adjust; prepare and embrace it—it lasts a long time.

References

19. Five Guide-Enhancing Caesarean section recovery. https://www.rcn.org.uk/celebrating-nursing-practice/janine-mcknight-cowan

20. SAC Splint—https://www.leonierastas.com/product/wearable-splint/

21. Lullaby Trust Safe Sleep—www.lullabytrust.org.uk

22. Retrieved from https://rednose.org.au/downloads/InfoStatement_SharingSleepSurfacewithBaby_Dec2019.pdf

23. Numerical Pain Score- National Center for Biotechnology Information, U.S. National Library of Medicine, Medscape, National Center for Biotechnology Information, U.S. National Library of Medicine

24. How to cope with stress—https://www.nhs.uk/oneyou/every-mind-matters/

25. Pelvic floor management—http://www.pelvicfloorfirst.org.au/pages

26. Postnatal exercise—https://www.babycentre.co.uk/x1960/when-can-i-exercise-after-a-caesarean

27. Swollen legs/complications—https://www.nhs.uk/conditions/pregnancy-and-baby/swollen-ankles-feet-pregnant/

Chapter 6
Mastering the art and skill of feeding baby

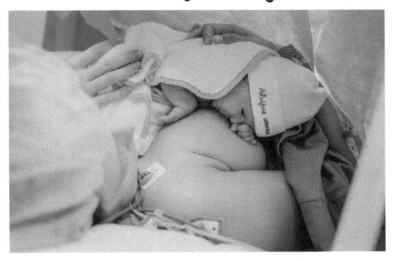

Why you should read this chapter:

- To understand the role of early skin-to-skin contact in successful breastfeeding.
- To understand that breastfeeding is both an art and physiological science.
- Breastfeeding, although considered natural, is still a learned skill for new mothers.
- To support your understanding of how a surgical birth might impact lactation.
- To learn the science of breastfeeding.
- To learn how mindset and confidence impact successful breastfeeding.
- To help give you the confidence to 'have a go'.
- To be mindful of the particular circumstances that require specialist support.
- If it is a decision to bottle feed, here are some top tips.

The practice of whisking babies away after a brief meeting with mum and dad has thankfully changed. Research has discovered the benefits of immediate skin-to-skin contact for both mother and baby at birth.

Skin-to-skin care (also called kangaroo care) is a natural process that involves placing a naked newborn on the mother's bare chest and covering the infant with blankets to keep it dry and warm. Ideally, skin-to-skin care starts immediately after birth or shortly after birth, with the baby remaining on the mother's chest until at least the end of the first breastfeeding session.[28]

6.1 Expressing Breastmilk

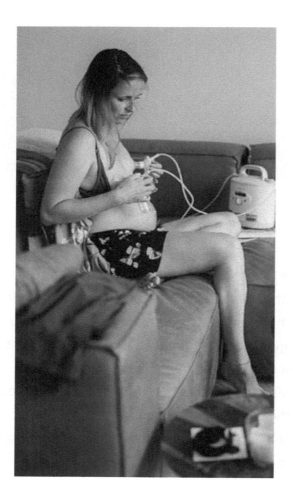

Leonie's Story

I remember the ache vividly in my heart at not being able to hold or see my babies until sometime later. I needed to get stitched up before I was eventually free to hold my baby, and then they were so tightly wrapped the only part visible was a portion of a tiny little face looking through the peephole. I had my first C-section back in 1980, at a time when babies seemed to belong to the hospital, guided by policy; they were stored in nurseries between feeds and only allowed out every four hours. Pity the poor babies who were missing their mums within the four hours; they would more often be settled with a drink of cow's milk formula or a pacifier to soothe them.

As a midwife of many decades, I have been part of the C-section production line in the operating theatre. I would wait to take the baby from the doctor, say a quick hello to mum and dad, and then busily do the routine checks and labelling while mum waited until she could have her first cuddle. I would see firsthand how the startled babies looked after being suddenly lifted out of their secure, warm wet environment to be passed to the waiting midwife who was holding a sterile cloth ready to transfer the baby to the resuscitation cot. The warmed crib had bright overhead lights for assessment and visibility should the baby need assistance breathing. Imagine that the newborn baby is one minute snug in his natural habitat, and next minute he is hurriedly being dried with a cloth and clothed in some strange wrapper. I do feel somewhat sad that none of my babies ever had the comfort of skin-to-skin cuddles immediately after birth, where they could hear my familiar heartbeat and experience warmth by my cuddle.

I am grateful for the research that has led to change today. I am thankful that in my clinical practice, I have been able to witness many beautiful caesarean births where mums have been able to engage in immediate skin-to-skin with their babies.

Research about early skin-to-skin contact for mothers and their healthy newborn infants is available through a Google search.

If you choose to breastfeed, it is helpful to build your understanding and skills antenatally. Seek out any courses for your partners as they can be a valuable source of support and encouragement.

Knowing that breastfeeding is both an art and a science and can take you a few weeks to feel confident and competent at feeding can help you to have realistic expectations. Some women find breastfeeding easy from the first feed, while others find hurdles along the way.

Help is available

Remember there are health professionals and community breastfeeding support groups who specialise in helping you master the art and skill to suit your needs.

Not all doctors, nurses, and midwives have the specialised training to offer ongoing mentoring for breastfeeding issues, so be sure to seek out an accredited lactation consultant in your area if you have problems.

In Australia and the UK, lactation consultants are also maternal and child health nurses, midwives, and health visitors who offer telephone support as well as face-to-face home visiting.

Australia and the UK have a comprehensive global partnership to support all new mothers to achieve breastfeeding, including the Australian Breastfeeding Association (ABA),[29] UNICEF's Baby-Friendly Hospital Initiative,[30] Lactation Consultants Australia & New Zealand,[31] and Lactation Consultants Great Britain.[32]

Getting breastfeeding started

The biological process that triggers your milk to 'come in' is the birth of the placenta. Your baby's frequent suckling and expressing milk will then build up your milk supply and help establish breastfeeding.

Skin-to-skin breast and chest contact as soon as possible after birth will help the baby to develop a sucking reflex that is usually present during the first hour after birth (in a well baby beyond thirty-five weeks' gestation).

Positioning the baby's hands circling the breast is helpful, as is placing the baby's chest to be in contact with your chest and nipple. The baby's nose should be at the nipple.

This position will help the baby's primitive instinct to latch and feed in the early days. There are multiple different feeding positions to feed in, but the best is the one that works for you, where your baby is getting milk, and it's pain-free.

If your baby needs extra care in the nursery, you may need to express some colostrum until the baby can be with you. Neonatal unit staff will discuss breastfeeding for prematurely born babies. In the unit, breastfeeding is encouraged due to its high nutritional value and protection against infection and diseases. If your baby is not yet strong enough to suckle, you will be offered support to express your milk and your milk will be fed via a small tube into the stomach.

Your comfort is one of the essential considerations when breastfeeding. You need to be in a relaxed position to avoid tension on your abdomen and stitches. It is also important to intentionally relax your shoulders to aid the letdown reflex. Muscle tension can cause a delay in letting milk down. Be mindful of how you're feeling in regard to the relaxation of your shoulders. Imagining your milking flowing may also help as you prepare to feed. Letdown is a hormonal response where hormones are released, and often women experience a tingling sensation in the breast.

Wound or wind pain can also inhibit let-down, so be sure you are pain-free with regular medication. It may be helpful to do some breathing exercises before you position yourself to feed to give yourself the best chance of reducing tension.

Comfortable position to adopt in the early postoperative days include:

- Side-lie on your bed, baby next to your breast, and your arm parallel with the pillow. Bring the baby to your nipple to feed.
- A pillow between your legs will ease the strain on your wound.
- Placing a towel or something soft in front of the scar to cushion the baby's feet kicking against the scar.

Figure 6.2 Side lying feeding. Smith, P. 2019

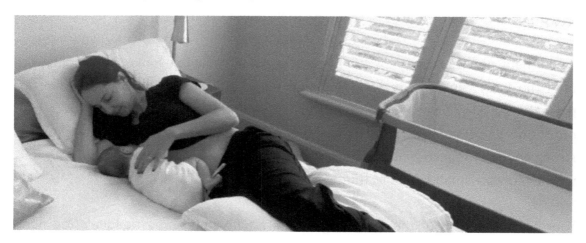

Let-down reflex

The let-down reflex is the description given to a feeling of milk ejection, at sucking or even earlier with experiencing baby cues like a baby's cry. Tiny nerves stimulate the nipple, which causes the hormone Oxytocin to release, or let down, the breast milk. Check out: <https://www.breastfeeding.asn.au/bf-info/early-days/let-down-reflex>.

Breastfeeding concerns and helpful strategies
I do not want to breastfeed

How you wish to feed your baby is your decision, and your reasons may be of a very personal nature that you don't want to discuss. Be sure to let your healthcare providers know. Your midwife, maternal and child health nurse, or health visitor will help you with either expressing breast milk, or formula feeding information. The choices of milk products are vast, and there will be lots of gimmicks and sales propaganda to get your interest. Our top tips are:

- Choose a formula with first steps nutritional advice.
- Read the bottle make up advice.
- Make sure your water temperature is correct—killing bacteria is vital.
- Sterilise your bottles efficiently, read the information on water, microwave, or electric sterilisers.
- Avoid making up bottles in advance—freshly made is recommended.
- If you are out and about, take a carton, or make up the milk fresh from a flask of hot water.
- Avoid too many people feeding the baby. Limit this activity to parents, initially.
- Bottle-feeding is paced and should be on-demand when the baby needs it, not on a timed basis.
- When travelling, consider hygiene and avoid gastroenteritis. Ready-made cartons are safer options at these times. Some bottled water is high in minerals and should be avoided.
- How much to give your baby depends on weight, age, and need.
- Stages and ages milk is not necessary if your baby is thriving.
- Always clean the pieces of a bottle independently. Remember, bacteria can grow in tiny crevices.
- Always add the water first, then the scoops of powder.
- Read up on your choice of product's website.

Bottle feeding, like breastfeeding, is still to be enjoyed—never rushed. Never leave a baby alone with a bottle; it can easily choke.

Check out further reading at <https://www.unicef.org.uk/babyfriendly/?s=bottle+-feeding>.

Expressing breast milk—how to store it and give it to your baby

Expressing breast milk manually or mechanically and feeding from a cup or bottle is an alternative way of breastfeeding your baby. In the early days postpartum, there are many things that can steer you away from skin-to-skin breastfeeding. These include pain, fatigue, ill health, and lack of confidence. It doesn't mean you cannot, with support, feed your baby your breast milk. Expressing breast milk comes in many forms, and the mum whose baby is in the neonatal unit will be encouraged to express her breast milk—possibly even more so than mothers on a postnatal unit or in the community. The term *expressing* breast milk means squeezing milk out of your breast so you can save or store it to feed your baby later. You may use a mechanical pump, hand-held pump, or your own hands to achieve this. However, it will give you time to decide and a few days of recovery thinking after a C-section. Especially useful to consider if your baby is unable to latch onto your breast initially. Milk flow is stimulated by having your baby near you and having a schedule that encourages milk production with regular expressing times scheduled within a twenty-four-hour period. Join the conversation on expressing and check out further reading at <https://www.nhs.uk/conditions/baby/breastfeeding-and-bottle-feeding/breastfeeding/expressing-breast-milk/> and <https://www.breastfeeding.asn.au/bf-info/breastfeeding-and-work/expressing-and-storing-breastmilk>.

I tried to feed a previous baby, but it did not work. Will I be able to do it?

Your previous breastfeeding experience is no indicator of how the next feeding experience will be. No two babies are the same, so if you would like to feed, it is certainly possible to have a positive outcome.

It hurts so much

Breastfeeding should not hurt. Get advice from your healthcare professional (HCPs), lactation consultants, or breastfeeding counsellors if it does. Don't suffer pain as you could cause severe nipple damage. Painful breastfeeding is most often due to a poor latch or sucks, even tongue-tie.

I have inverted nipples

Inverted nipples can make breastfeeding a challenge. But it is not impossible to feed. There are products available to buy online to support nipple inversion.

I have breast implants

Breastfeeding with implants is achievable. It is sometimes a little more uncomfortable, and it can also affect a mother's ability to produce a full milk supply. Check out <https://www.whattoexpect.com/first-year/breastfeeding-with-implants> and <https://www.breastfeeding.asn.au/bfinfo/breastfeeding-after-breast-surgery>.

Can I only give the colostrum feed?

You choose how much or little you want to feed your baby; if you only wish to feed the colostrum, it's your choice.

Check out the benefits of colostrum:

<https://www.bellybelly.com.au/breastfeeding/colostrum/>

Will I get support?

Yes, there is help available. Speak with your maternity support team and ask for a referral to the best option for you. If your baby is crying and you need assistance, you call for your help too.

Australian Resource <https://www.breastfeeding.asn.au/breastfeeding-helpline>

UK Resource <https://www.nhs.uk/conditions/baby/breastfeeding-and-bottle-feeding/breastfeeding/help-and-support/>

What is mastitis?

Mastitis is a condition where your milk ducts in the breast become inflamed, often referred to as 'milk fever'. It is caused by a blocked milk duct that does not clear. The banked-up milk behind the blocked duct is then forced into the nearby breast tissue, causing the tissue to become inflamed. Infection may or may not be present.

If you think you have mastitis, continue to feed and consult your doctor. Antibiotics may be needed if it becomes infected.

What are the symptoms?
- Pain
- Engorgement
- Hot breast
- Swelling/lump at the site
- High temperature
- Feeling unwell
- Red area sore to touch.

Early symptoms of mastitis can make you feel as if you are getting the flu. You may begin to get shivers and aches.

Initial treatment
- Pain relief
- Anti-inflammatory (if prescribed)
- Continue to breastfeed your baby
- Seek medical advice.[33]

What if I just can't do it?
That's okay! You are not alone; you tried, and that's great. However, if you are not ready to give up, get help!

Australian Resource: <https://www.breastfeeding.asn.au/breastfeeding-helpline>

UK Resource: <https://www.nhs.uk/conditions/baby/breastfeeding-and-bottle-feeding/breastfeeding/help-and-support/>

Can I dual feed with breast and bottle?
Yes. Dual feeding is quite regular in many cultures and is common with multiple pregnancies. Breast and bottle feeding can be sufficient to suit the mother's needs.[34]

Feeding in public

You may feel self-conscious feeding in public; however, there are a variety of capes and shawls that you can use to feed discreetly. Many venues offer feeding areas signposted by universal symbols. Many shopping centres and public buildings have feeding rooms if you prefer.

UK: <https://www.unicef.org.uk/babyfriendly/about/breastfeeding-in-the-uk/>

Australia: <https://www.breastfeeding.asn.au/babycarerooms/list>

What if I just don't like the feeling or it feels 'yuk'?

You don't have to continue. Listen to your body; if it triggers an unpleasant reaction in you, then stop. It's okay to do what you need to do.

What is 'tongue-tie'?

Tongue-tie occurs when the thin membrane under the baby's tongue (called the lingual frenulum) restricts the movement of the tongue. In some cases, the tongue is not free or mobile enough for the baby to attach properly to the breast. Tongue-tie occurs in 4–11% of newborns and is more common in males.[35]

While some babies feed efficiently with a tongue-tie, some will need a surgical procedure to address possible problems associated, such as nipple pain and damage, flattening of the nipple, compression marks on the nipple, and baby failing to gain weight.

Speak with your HCP if you suspect tongue-tie. In most countries, it can be surgically snipped.

Can I freeze expressed breast milk?

Yes. Equipment needs to be sterilised, and you must wash your hands thoroughly beforehand. Freezing breast milk can be a lifesaver when you need an early night; your partner or helper can heat it and feed your baby. Check with your local breastfeeding authority for evidence-based best practices in technique, timing, and thawing.

Remember to:

- Freeze small amounts and leave a space at the top of the container as it expands when frozen.
- Date it/label it.
- Defrost in the fridge and use within 12 hours.
- Warm up in the bottle in a bowl of warm water and gently rotate.
- Never heat in a pan or the microwave.

If breast milk is left standing, the fat will separate and rise to the top. Gently swirl to remix.[36]

Australian Resource: <https://raisingchildren.net.au/babies/breastfeeding-bottle-feeding-solids/expressing-working-travelling/expressing-breastmilk>

UK Resource: https://www.nhs.uk/conditions/baby/breastfeeding-and-bottle-feeding/breastfeeding/expressing-breast-milk/

How do I know if I have enough milk?

You can tell if a baby is having enough milk by looking for the number of wet nappies; up to six wet nappies in twenty-four hours is a good indicator. The baby will be alert and reasonably contented after feeds also. A breastfed baby's urine should be pale. They will often poop even at each feed.

Weight monitoring in the early weeks gives reassurance that your baby is absorbing calories and growing.[37]

What if my milk supply seems low?

Galactagogues are foods like fennel and fenugreek, herbs, or medications that can help to increase breast milk supply, for example, whole grains, dark leafy greens, papaya, and chickpeas. The use of a galactagogue to help improve low breast milk supply requires consultation with a lactation consultant and medical adviser.

Australia: https://raisingchildren.net.au/newborns/breastfeeding-bottle-feeding/breastfeeding-challenges/increase-supply

UK: https://www.laleche.org.uk/my-baby-needs-more-milk/

How do I know when the baby is ready to breastfeed?

Whenever your baby is showing feeding cues—sticking their tongue out or turning their head from side to side, crying, trying to nurture—these are indicators that your baby is ready to feed.[38]

Why are my nipples sore?

It is quite reasonable for nipples to be tender in the early first few days of breastfeeding, but they will get better. Sometimes smearing a little breast milk after each feed and allowing them to air dry can help. It is more relaxed at home to air dry in privacy, but in the hospital, an easy way to air your nipples privately is to position your bed table so the sheet drapes over the top while you lay in bed. Do not ignore sore nipples; seek advice as it is often a result of poor attachment at suckling.[39]

How can I tell if my baby is feeding well?

You can tell your baby is feeding well when you see his jaw and possibly his face muscles and tips of his ears are moving. You will probably hear him suck and swallow. Signs include wet nappies, dirty nappies, quiet periods between feeds, and weight gain.

It should not be painful to breastfeed your baby; any nipple soreness is likely due to an incorrect attachment to the breast.

How often do I need to feed my baby?

Young babies need to feed often; it is common for a baby to feed eight to twelve times in twenty-four hours, though some may need to feed ten to fifteen times or as few as six to eight times within that period. You cannot overfeed a breastfed baby; they are born with the instinct to know when they have had enough to match their bodies.

Feeding patterns change, and rarely are two days the same. Responsive or on-demand feeding is recommended by most experts in the field.

I have a hard lump in my breast—what is that?

Sometimes the breast can develop a blocked duct, which presents as a hard, painful lump. It may even be associated with redness and a mild fever. To clear the blockage, gentle massage toward the nipple while feeding or in the shower can help remove it. If this does not disappear and is troubling you, seek medical advice.

What if I have to return to work and I am still breastfeeding?

Breastfeeding can continue; there is a range of options:

- Expressing at work and feeding the expressed milk.
- Having a baby in childcare nearby or working from home.
- Giving bottles when you cannot be present.
- Consider your storage options/fridge, etc.
- Talk to your employer about returning to work as a breastfeeder.

You do have rights; ask your employer about their breastfeeding policy.

What if I don't want my baby to have a bottle?

Babies can be successfully cup fed. The cup is positioned at the bottom lip and the milk should be gently lapped from the edge, thereby controlling the volume of fluid taken into the mouth. This method needs careful technique so as to not overpour and overwhelm the baby.

Why is my baby not gaining weight like my friends' babies?

Breastfed babies can have different weight gain patterns from formula-fed babies. Speak to your HCP if you are concerned, but remember weight gain is only one indicator of healthy development.

What is the best position for breastfeeding a baby?

There is no one 'best' position. It should feel comfortable and should not hurt. There are many different positions, so whatever works for you is best, though, for C-section mums, the side-lying on the bed position is worth trying.[40]

Baby should get a good mouthful of breast quickly with his mouth wide open and lips turned outward, especially the lower lip. Check the baby's head is tilted back so that the chin is well against your breast, and the nose is free to breathe without your fingers helping.

Check out <https://www.nhs.uk/conditions/pregnancy-and-baby/breastfeeding-positioning-attachment/> and see Dr Jack Newman's YouTube guides: <https://www.youtube.com/watch?v=56YzjsZr4hQ>.

Neck pain while breastfeeding

When breastfeeding, sit comfortably. Try a pillow under your baby on your lap for support. Try to switch between watching the baby and looking up so your neck doesn't get too sore. You can also try feeding the baby while lying on your side.

Check out this video: <https://www.youtube.com/watch?v=X0JsX2K3FjA>

Does a baby need vitamin supplements when breastfeeding?

Research has confirmed the practice of vitamin D supplementation for term breastfed infants can prevent vitamin D deficiency and improve bone health—the reason being that vitamin D levels are low in breast milk, and babies often have limited exposure to sunlight. The recommended dose for vitamin D supplementation of infants is between 8.5–10 micrograms daily starting from birth up till one year of age and given via pipette dropper. You can purchase vitamin D drops from nearly any pharmacy or grocery store. Formula-fed babies will usually find formulas containing added vitamin D.

Check out more on vitamin D:

UK: <https://www.nhs.uk/start4life/baby/breastfeeding/healthy-diet/vitamins-for-mum-and-baby/>

Australia: <https://raisingchildren.net.au/teens/healthy-lifestyle/nutrients/vitamin-d>

Dietary intake during breastfeeding

If you are breastfeeding, you will burn more calories—at least 500–700 calories or 2092–2928 kJ daily.

Feeding longer has positive health benefits for you both.

Try to avoid any health problems that could be diet-related; it is best to avoid some foods like:

- Atlantic cod
- spicy foods
- prawns
- honey
- garlic
- chocolate
- strawberry
- pineapple
- cherries
- alcohol
- excessive dairy products.

Eating a healthy diet includes advice on rest, vitamins, and fluid intake. Check out:

<https://www.nhs.uk/conditions/pregnancy-and-baby/breastfeeding-diet/> and <https://www.betterhealth.vic.gov.au/health/HealthyLiving/breastfeeding-and-your-diet>.

Fluid intake while breastfeeding

Staying hydrated while breastfeeding is vital. Always have some water with you as you will likely experience thirst while feeding. A habit of drinking at least a glass of water/ juice at each breast-feed is a good tip—when a baby drinks, mamma drinks.

Check out: <https://www.verywellfamily.com/does-drinking-more-water-affect-breast-feeding-284285> and <https://raisingchildren.net.au/guides/first-1000-days/looking-after-yourself/breastfeeding-diet-lifestyle>.

Rest and breastfeeding

Tiredness and fatigue and learning to become a breastfeeder go hand in hand.

Some even find it so exhausting they want to give up. So, be patient, pace yourself, and nurture the time to learn this skill and art. Sleep when the baby sleeps and recover in between the feeding sessions you experience in the early weeks.

Afternoon power naps and recovery is what we are about with this journal. Lots of things that will make you tired go hand in hand with feeding, recovering, healing, parenting, caring, etc. Pace yourself.

Check out: <https://www.medela.com/breastfeeding/mums-journey/support-first-month> and <https://www.breastfeeding.asn.au/bf-info/you-and-your-breastfed-baby/yourself>

Maternity Bras

D, DD+, and EE+ sizes are practical and often required in the early weeks of establishing breastfeeding. Getting measured after your milk has come in is also a good idea, as you cannot envisage how much your breasts can grow.

The type of fabric, shape, and strapping will be your choice.

It is unclear whether wearing a bra does prevent stretch marks, but you will struggle to get into your pre-breastfeeding bras once your milk has come in.

You choose whether or not to wear a maternity bra. However, women with larger breasts may be more comfortable. It is a good idea to get professionally fitted, if possible. Underwire bras can block milk ducts and cause mastitis, as can individual styles with flaps that tighten when breasts are full. Breast size will fluctuate as you establish feeding.

Check out: <https://www.nct.org.uk/pregnancy/worries-and-discomforts/common-discomforts/maternity-bras-and-nursing-bras-what-you-need-know> and <https://www.breastfeeding.asn.au/bf-info/your-baby-arrives/choosing-maternity-bra>.

Support and comfort are key: your breasts will become heavy and can leak in the early weeks.

Summary

Breastfeeding can be a challenge, so ensure you celebrate and share the rewards of your success. We all know that breastfeeding is best as you pass on antibodies to your baby to help them fight off infections and disease, plus, it's free and readily available, amongst many other benefits.[41] Breastfeeding, however, requires a lot of effort, and that's not just from a mamma.

Those around you can also support you in the early weeks: your partner, your mother, a grandmother, a friend, or even a breastfeeding support specialist. All have a part to play in 'getting you going' and keeping you there.

So, whether or not it's your first baby or your first C-section, you have a lot on your plate; share it, get help, seek support, and nurture another role you have since becoming a mother.

Remember, your body is healing, repairing, and making milk!

Consider who is your breastfeeding family for support.

Breastfeeding offers benefits for both mother and baby; however, for many women, it is not an option. Your decision about how you will be feeding your baby should be respected and supported.

While breastfeeding is a natural process, it does not always come naturally, and one-on-one mentoring may be needed. Lactation consultants throughout the world provide a range of personal and group services. The Australian Breastfeeding Association is Australia's peak breastfeeding support group providing trained counsellors and mother-to-mother support.

Throughout the chapter, we have signposted to several respected websites and video links. They can all support you in your journey to become a successful breastfeeder or even an expressing breastfeeder. But you need to nurture and care for yourself also, so you can be the breastfeeder mamma you want to be.

Remember, breastfeeding and formula feeding both benefit the baby; a healthy food source is a responsible parenting choice.

If you need to talk to someone about your experiences, anything, make that call, and seek support.

Remember, you are not alone!

References

28. Dekker, R (2017) Evidence on Skin-to- skin After Cesarean. Retrieved from https://evidencebasedbirth.com/the-evidence-for-skin-to-skin-care-after-a-cesarean/

29. From https://www.breastfeeding.asn.au/

30. From https://sites.unicef.org/nutrition/index_24806.html

31. From https://www.lcanz.org/find-a-lactation-consultant/

32. From https://lcgb.org/

33. From https://www.nhs.uk/conditions/mastitis/

34. From https://www.nhs.uk/conditions/pregnancy-and-baby/combining-breast-and-bottle/

35. From https://www.breastfeeding.asn.au/bf-info/tongue-tie

36. From https://www.laleche.org.uk/storing-your-milk/; https://www.nhs.uk/conditions/pregnancy-and-baby/express-ing-storing-breast-milk/

37. From https://www.nhs.uk/conditions/pregnancy-and-baby/breastfeeding-is-baby-getting-enough-milk/; https://www.llli.org/breastfeeding-info/is-baby-getting-enough/

38. From https://www.llli.org/breastfeeding-info/frequency-feeding-frequently-asked-questions-faqs/

39. From https://www.nhs.uk/conditions/baby/breastfeeding-and-bottle-feeding/breastfeeding-problems/sore-nipples/

40. From https://www.babycentre.co.uk/a8784/good-positions-for-breastfeeding

41. From https://www.healthline.com/health/breastfeeding/11-benefits-of-breastfeeding#benefits-for-baby

Chapter 7
Safe sleeping and managing a crying baby

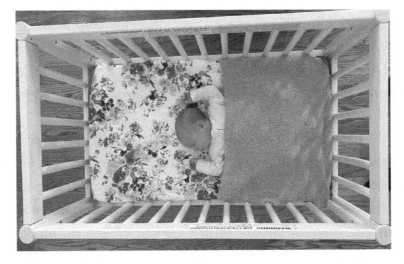

Why you should read this chapter:

- To learn about safe sleeping practices.
- To understand sleep deprivation and survival strategies.
- To learn the impact of sleep deprivation on physical and mental health.
- Understand how sleep deprivation can affect your coping mechanisms.
- To learn how to understand a baby's cry.

Figure 7.1 Safe Sleeping

This is a well-researched document from 'The Red Nose Foundation' in Australia about the risks of sleep accidents: <https://rednose.org.au/article/bedding-amount-recommended-for-safe-sleep1>.

> Newborn babies can burst the bubble of glitter and magic when it comes to your sleep.
>
> —Janine

What is sleep deprivation?

Sleep deprivation, also known as insufficient sleep. It is often an acute consequence of the birth of a new baby. Fatigue is inevitable in the early days and weeks postpartum, with the baby requiring round-the-clock attention while your body is repairing after major surgery. We recommend realistic planning to help prevent fatigue from becoming overwhelming. As midwives, mothers, and grandmothers, we would both agree that sleep deprivation is one of the leading causes of maternal and parenting distress.

Sleeping when the baby sleeps is, of course, ideal and one of our top recommendations; however, the practicalities of that will depend on the gestation of your baby, whether there are any siblings, your birth experience, and the support network you can set up around yourself. This chapter is one of the most important for validating why you need that 'afternoon nap' or snooze on the couch. Broken or interrupted sleep by night feeding disrupts the natural sleep rhythm, leaving you feeling sleep-deprived as if you'd just had four hours rest a night. It may mean you do not reach the most therapeutic, deeper phases of sleep. Many say that two hours sleep before midnight is worth four hours after midnight!

While there is no magic cure other than getting a night nanny, training yourself into a sleep regime where you can catch up on lost sleep is vital.

Schedule naps on your planner; you won't need a reason after you know why sleep deprivation is a problem for you, your baby, and your recovery.

There are many useful and popular websites on sleep management, safe sleep, and coping strategies; for example: <https://www.breastfeeding.asn.au/bfinfo/how-cope-broken-sleep>.

What, why, and how you can resolve sleep issues

This section will identify frequently asked questions about sleep, why it is a problem, and some ideas to make it easier.

How long should a baby sleep?

Sleep and your newborn baby will vary day by day. The problem is your baby will sleep when they need to, and there will be no pattern or length. It purely will depend on feeding needs initially. Ideally, a newborn to six weeks old should need to sleep between fourteen to seventeen hours a day.

Feed your baby milk on demand. Responsive feeding is the key; a baby does not have any sense of time, hours, or routine. They are independent; each baby will have its own needs. Even twins or multiples may have different sleep patterns.

Keep the baby clean, warm, and fed, and give them a healthy mix of social interaction; rest and recovery are crucial to developing the confidence to understand your baby's needs.

Two popular resources available in Australia are the Australian Breastfeeding Association and the Raising Children Network supported by the Australian Government Social services.

1. <https://www.breastfeeding.asn.au/bf-info/sleep/wakeful>
2. <https://raisingchildren.net.au/newborns/sleep/understanding-sleep/newborn-sleep>

Why can't I cope with simple things?

Sleep deprivation will influence your coping mechanisms. Daily routines, tasks, and activities you usually dealt well with are affected by lack of sleep.

You can improve this by eating well and drinking plenty of fresh fluids. But also read your body's need to rest, recover, and recuperate. Everyone will react differently to sleep loss; it can cause a chemical imbalance and lead to stress reactions. Take that afternoon nap every day where practical for your postpartum period.

I feel guilty falling asleep
The human body needs sleep to help prevent burnout.

A baby will sleep to grow, so just like your baby, you need to sleep to recover.

You will rejuvenate all your cells and tissues to withstand the early weeks of recovery and parenting. Don't continue to be consumed with any feelings of guilt; they serve no purpose for your emotional and spiritual wellbeing. Seek professional help if necessary.

I do not have enough help
A newborn baby is a social magnet for you to call on friends and family to support you. Engaging a handful of support networks around you will require you to think about how you will cope.

Without a support network, you only have yourself to rely upon, and you will be unable to juggle all the skills and jobs required to care for yourself and your baby.

Try to let go feelings of guilt by asking for help. It is, in fact, a sign of positive parenting and personal care planning to set this support network up as soon as you can pre- or post-surgery; you can soon make them redundant once you are well enough to do things again yourself.

Some more helpful advice can be found on Australia's Raising Children Network website: <https://raisingchildren.net.au/pregnancy/labour-birth/recovery-after-birth/after-caesarean>.

Be mindful not to take on extra responsibilities and jobs
Saying 'no', 'I can't', and 'I won't be' is hard for some women who say yes to doing everything. Try buying time and saying 'let me get back to you'.

Finishing your job, worrying if the nursery is finished, or keeping the home as clean and sorted as you always have need careful thought.

Having a caesarean section and a new baby to care for will force you to make realistic coping choices that can soon fatigue and tire you beyond any household chore or employment role ever did.

Doing the best job you can as a mum and recovering the best way you can as a C-section mum is for you to decide.

Your body and your recovery involve the need for sleep, rest, and healing as part of your plan, just like food, fluids, medication, and wound recovery.

Should I suggest that my partner and I do sleep shifts?
Humans are not supposed to be sleep-deprived. You are taking it in turns, hopefully, to feed a baby if bottle-fed. But if you are recovering from a C-section and breastfeeding, the scales are already in your favour. Physical recovery and then learning to breastfeed takes an enormous number of calories a day. You need to be the one getting more sleep, more rest, and less in the way of being sleep-deprived with shift patterns.

Sleep as much as you can; you are healing and, if breastfeeding, making milk to feed your baby. It is a good idea to share roles, depending on the task. While night-time awakenings will be the most distressing, catching up on sleep in the day is a gift to be enjoyed. Subtle sharing about how poorly you feel when doing certain tasks may help you avoid the negativity of guilt in asking in the first place. Watching the Five Guide Video[42] may remove any hesitation from a loved one or support network in supporting you to recover. This video, in our experience, has enhanced the mother's support as it easily explains what surgery you have had and why you need help.

Without sustained support, your postpartum recovery will take its toll and last much longer than six weeks. Plan, ask for help, and allow your recovery to be supported.

My baby feeds a lot. What is responsive feeding?

Responsive feeding involves the mother's responses to the baby's feeding cues, such as crying or not sleeping. Responsive breastfeeding is the timely preparation and giving of a breastfeed or bottle that benefits both baby and mother. Responsive feeding is not time-controlled or based on how long since your baby was last fed. It is the natural reaction to a new baby's natural ability to wake, feed, and regulate their own need and intake of calories. Mothers, in turn, can also be relaxing, resting, and sleeping in between these events. Breastfed babies can feed up to twelve times a day.

My partner can sleep. Why can't I?

While you are trying to work as a team, your partner will just not tune in with the innate maternal protective instincts that usually come with motherhood.

Do not forget your body has been preparing itself for these changes during pregnancy. Even the reason you probably used to lie in a different position to get to sleep has now changed. Nine months of careful body positioning, hormonal changes, bladder disturbances, alongside a growing abdomen, all lead up to your C-section.

Those changes account for understanding why your slumber is compromised and not theirs. Your lack of sleep after C-section and birth is quite naturally going to be compounded by pain, discomfort, role expectations, breastfeeding, baby care, and exhaustion. Listen to yourself, and ask for help. Not short term; make it a postpartum plan that fits with your recovery plan. Try to avoid argument and negative communication—be open, honest, and realistic, and remember that you have the Five Guide video as a reminder for non-engaging partners.

How can I get my partner to help out more?

Relationships can take a considerable dip after a baby is born, and especially after a C-section. When one person feels they are not able to share the burden and load of new work and roles, it can lead to conflict. We all want our partners to be more responsive. But we need to ask, delegate, or formulate a list of chores to support the recovery plan.

Being done asking is not the answer; change the tactic. Five Guide videos will help to explain your surgery and why you need more help to recover.

If you are just not getting the help you need, end the chore war with a good bucket of tears. Then source a new network of willing helpers.

—Janine

Simon's story

Our baby was born by C-section after a long labour. Gabby said she found the following tips to be very helpful. Breastfeeding made Gabby very thirsty, so I made it my job to always keep her drink bottle filled up during feed time. At night, I got up with her for the night feeds, as it can be a lonely place and I wanted her to feel supported. After a few weeks, Gabby told me when she felt comfortable to feed alone during the night. I made sure there was a stack of clean towels next to her feeding chair in case baby Ollie spilt his feeds. I shared the nappy changing with Gabby and found it wasn't as scary as I thought; and I thought it was the least I could do as I hadn't had to go through 9 months of carrying the baby! Ollie was born during COVID-19 pandemic, so I worked from home, which meant I was able to help Gabby with any heavy lifting or strenuous housework. One final word of warning: 'day three blues' are a thing, so I made sure to be extra caring during that time as Gabby was very emotional.

Why am I so grumpy?

There is science behind being cranky and grumpy. Sleep deprivation, ill health, anaemia, and a poor diet can all lead to why you may feel like you do.

When we feel irritable, it is an emotional state we experience. How we get ourselves out of it is the key.

'Baby blues' and postpartum depression observations can include symptoms of forgetfulness, anxiety, inadequate coping mechanisms, and grumpy, flat, emotional, or high alert and manic states.

If you are concerned about your mood and after sleep or recovery time, you still feel down, it is important to share your feelings with your partner or trusted friend, and if there is no improvement, reach out to your healthcare professional.

The baby blues often occurs after arriving home, with periods of crying followed by periods of joy that seem to come from nowhere. It is a common response and is related to the hormonal changes you experience following birth.

I feel very stressed when my baby cries
If your baby's cry stirs up a feeling of anxiety and panic within you or your partner, you are not alone! A baby's cry can be a similar pitch and volume as a police siren. Both evoke panic and stress. How you respond to the cry is critical.

Be calm, be safe, be methodical. A baby's cry is their only way of communicating to you that they need something. They may need feeding, changing, or burping. Just be gentle, caring, and protective. Remember, they can't tell you what they need, and they are only trying to communicate with you. If you are distressed by the crying, get help, take time out, make a hot drink, and come back to the baby when you are calm. Getting what it needs is often trial and error.

Sadly, babies can suffer severe brain trauma if shaken when they cry. Never shake a baby; you could seriously damage them, or at worst, cause a fatality! If you cannot cope, tell someone. Asking for help is a sign of good parenting. Some useful tips for unsettled babies can be found on Australia's Centre of Parenting Excellence website: <https://www.cope.org.au/new-parents/first-weeks/coping-with-an-unsettled-baby/>.

Figure 7.2 Stop That Shake Babies Break!
<https://www.youtube.com/watch?v=TMyCrKPa6Gl>.

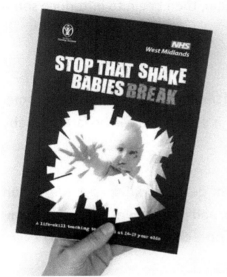

Is sleep deprivation linked to postpartum depression (PPD)?

In our experience, almost all new parents experience sleep deprivation and complete exhaustion at some point. But, in postpartum depression, which affects approximately one in seven parents, it's quality more than the quantity of sleep that's the problem, with PPD sufferers reporting that they simply don't sleep well as they are often disturbed by anxiety and ruminating thoughts.

Measure your mood, observe your sleep pattern, and look at what you eat and drink to assess your attachment to your baby and your ability to evaluate and enjoy your baby and your new life.

Health professionals have many ways of assessing mood and monitoring for PPD.

If you think you may be suffering from PPD, talk with your doctor right away. There are successful ways to treat the condition, and the vast majority of parents can gain control of their situation, allowing them to experience all the joys—albeit sleep-deprived ones—of life with a new baby.

My baby won't sleep

Hey, your baby is also adjusting to life outside of the womb. Depending on birth history and wellbeing, babies who do not appear to sleep will soon improve.

Your baby doesn't know if it is night or day, breakfast time, or suppertime. So, to meet the demands of your baby, you may need to change your sleep patterns to fit theirs.

While they might initially sleep both day and night, eventually, by three–four months, their pattern of sleep will begin to match a night and day pattern.

You cannot force sleep on a baby, meet its needs again, then begin to introduce some baby playtime to stimulate them gently.[43]

What is shaken baby syndrome?

Shaken baby syndrome—also known as abusive head trauma, shaken impact syndrome, inflicted head injury, or non-accidental head injury—is severe and can be fatal if a baby is shaken.[44]

Abusive head trauma is one of the leading causes of death in babies aged less than one year. If baby is inconsolable, walk away, get help, and calm down! Leave the room, make a hot drink, relax and drink it, pop the radio on—check in on your baby every five to ten minutes.

Only when you feel calmer and in control should you return to your baby. Try these techniques:

- **Walk away.**
- **Move your body.** Ease up, relax your shoulders.
- **Breathe deeply.** Take a few deep breaths in and out; relax.
- **Make time for yourself.** Make a hot drink sit and relax for a while.
- **Smile.** Tell yourself this is normal, it will pass, and you will try to learn a new coping skill.
- **Keep a journal.** Express your thoughts privately in your journal and get things off your chest. Drawing, sketching, and doodling can also help externalise and untangle your thoughts.
- **Call a friend.** You are not alone. Calling a friend allows you to vent when you get frustrated.
- **Ask for help.** Remember, it is a sign of good parenting.

How will eating and drinking fluids help my sleep?
A proper hydration and calorie schedule will support your sleep and recovery needs. It aids digestion and releases sugar and salts required to give you a positive nutrient balance for healing and recovery.

There are many surprising ways to reduce the interruption of sleep when in recovery. Dehydration can cause night-time leg cramps; drinking enough fluids can support body digestion and aid recovery.

Hunger can keep you awake, and if you are breastfeeding, you will use up to 500 more calories/2092KJ daily to make breast milk.

Consuming less than 1500 calories/6276KJ after surgery will not support your postnatal surgical recovery.

In addition to this, if you are breastfeeding, you need to upgrade your calorie intake by at least another 500 calories/2092KJ to support rest, recovery and sleep, and breast milk formulation.

If you are consuming any less than these amounts, it will put your recovery and milk production at risk.

Why can anaemia affect my sleep pattern?
Having low blood iron levels, known as iron deficiency post-C-section, will affect your sleep patterns—symptoms of iron deficiency is drowsiness. The body reacts to try to conserve energy for cell regeneration, fighting off an infection, or merely making breast milk. Fatigue and sleepiness go hand in hand with low blood count anaemia.

Up to one in five women can suffer from iron deficiency anaemia after having a baby.

If you feel tired all the time and have not been prescribed medication, seek medical advice.

However, you should take any prescribed anaemia medication to restore low iron levels.

When your body wants to conserve energy, iron deficiency will make you more tired.

Why should I never be in bed with my baby?
Never sleep with your baby on a sofa or armchair; this can increase the incidence of sudden infant death syndrome (SIDS).[45] If you are breastfeeding your baby, some positions after a C-section can help you to breastfeed lying down.

Co-sleeping is now not advised as it increases the likelihood of infant suffocation. Bed clothing, body heat, and the risk of rolling onto your baby are all increased if you bed-share. Babies should sleep in their own safe space, ideally in a crib/cot at the side of your bed, safely in the same room as their parents for at least six months.

They should sleep on their back at the foot of the crib, with no head supports or bedding too heavy to prevent them from moving safely in the crib.

Avoid letting pets into the sleeping area of a new baby.

It is essential to make sure that your baby's room is a comfortable temperature—not too hot or too cold. The chance of SIDS is higher in babies who get too hot, so try to keep the room temperature between 16–20°C.

How else can I relax?
It is easy to say 'relax' after you have just had a surgical birth, but in reality, it is one of the most challenging things to do as a new mother, especially after a C-section.

Is pain stopping you from sleeping? Pain will contribute to your inability to relax, and the techniques you choose to deal with pain management are important to your sleep.

Preserving your energy can be very different after a C-section, due to your ability to perform relaxing techniques like yoga or breathing exercises.

Yoga breathing can improve wellbeing, but any physical activities are not advised for a while. Getting rid of the stress might prove difficult with a new baby crying, demanding your attention almost twenty-four hours of your day.

Techniques we suggest to improve relaxation include:

- Enjoy some alone time.
- Read your recovery manual—log your feelings and record your journey in your daily planners.
- Write in your journal your baby birth story, your achievements, and your aims.
- Close your eyes and practice some breathing techniques.
- Take a power nap—sleep when your baby sleeps.
- Try some foot exercises: bend your toes, rotate your ankles, ask for a leg massage.
- Take a warm bath and ask not to be disturbed for a fixed time.
- Listen to some relaxing music.
- Spend some controlled time with family, friends, girlfriends, and your pet!
- Use any hypnobirthing techniques you may have learned antenatally.
- Mindful self-compassion meditation exercises.

Relaxing after surgery allows blood flow and increases oxygen levels to enhance tissue recovery and cell regeneration.

Deep breathing exercises relax the abdominal muscles and focus on sending signals of calm to your inner body.

Make sure any technique you choose is not too strenuous on you; remember, you are recovering.

Why can't I get back to sleep after feeding my baby?
Getting yourself back to sleep after feeding your baby is not so easy.

Baby will need night feeds, and you will naturally be learning to do without the much-needed sleep you may have enjoyed previously.

Trying to get back into a deep sleep will be an alert for your mind to start thinking again: thinking about all the things you need to do tomorrow, the next feed, the next cry, and the next tiring aching movement to change, bathe, and support not only your baby but for yourself.

It will mean you probably need to urinate and will be thirsty or hungry when all you want to do is sleep. You won't win initially! No baby is like a mythical unicorn who wakes just once in the night. Postpartum insomnia is real![46]

Routines for you and your baby take weeks to establish.

Tune into your little one's grunts and huffs; they are noises that will also keep you awake, you will soon learn to understand which is an 'I need you' noise.

Sleep during the day—play catch-up on your sleep. Cluster sleep as much as you can in the early weeks to support your postpartum insomnia. Whatever form it takes, do not let it impede your adjustment to recovery and motherhood.

Can my baby pick up on my feelings?
Your baby can pick up on the tone of your voice, body language, and facial expressions. Emotions are contagious; we know when we are happy, sad, or exhausted, we reflect these feelings in our words, behaviour, and facial expressions.

The first sign your baby will give you that you are connected and you are doing a good job is that first smile! But that won't come for at least five to eight weeks.

So, your baby will learn to mirror your emotions.

From birth, a baby picks up on emotional cues from others. Experimental research has confirmed that babies do pick up on stress.[47]

When you hear someone say, 'she has your strong personality,' it is a reflection of cues you are picking up from your baby, and your baby in turn with you. Shriek-cries happen, and your baby might not quickly calm. It is how you react and calm the situation that matters.

Spikes in your anxiety levels and how you deal with those situations will depend upon sleep, relaxation, pain relief, and whether you are eating well, have enough help and support, and are feeling anxious and depressed.

The nest you create for a baby in your home and post C-section surgery does collapse like a pack of cards now and then.

—Janine

What is fatigue?
Fatigue begins at birth, bringing with it all the emotional, physical, and social demands on the body, so don't be surprised by the onset of your fatigue. The key to managing your fatigue is to be responsive to signs of fatigue and rest to promote healing and recovery. You may find yourself overwhelmingly exhausted by the relentless demands of a new baby and managing a household and adjusting to the role of being responsible for your tiny new baby. Just know you are not alone; many mothers experience this, and it is where you may need help from family and friends to care for the baby and household for you while you rest.

You have good reason to feel fatigued after your baby's arrival and for the postpartum period, so tell yourself it is okay to feel tired.

There are many different types and causes and solutions for fatigue
Decision fatigue
It can be challenging to arrive at a decision when you are feeling mentally foggy from sleep deprivation. It may help to write a list of pros and cons relating to the issue and give each a score out of ten to arrive at a more considered decision.

Birth recovery
Your body is busy repairing from birth, and this takes energy to accomplish. Carrying a baby for nine months and then having major surgery is reason enough to feel fatigued.

Listen to your body without judgment and take time to rest or power nap when you feel depleted.

Anaemia

Blood loss greater than 500 mL during childbirth can cause temporary iron deficiency anaemia. A diet rich in iron will help restore balance. Be sure to also eat foods or drinks high in vitamin C, as iron needs vitamin C for effective absorption.

You may have been prescribed anaemia medication; please take it to support your recovery.

Poor self-care

When you feel tired or depressed, self-care can sometimes be unachievable.

Self-neglect impacts on meeting your basic needs, like washing, bathing, eating, dressing.

Whether you are aware you are doing it or not, taking care of yourself and hygiene is a vital part of your recovery.

Share how you feel with your support network. Ask for help, and it is a sign of good self-care.

Sleep needs for new mothers

On average, you will be lucky with just four hours each night. Do not fall victim and become sleep-fatigued. Please read the top tips on sharing the care of your baby, power napping, and sleeping when your baby sleeps.

Those top tips will help you to become less sleep-deprived.

Multitasking

Multitasking seems like a great idea. But not when you have a new baby or had a C-section!

Keep a task list and keep it simple. Delegate. Avoid over-thinking chores and tasks you would typically have done yourself.

Workload
What needs attention today?

Washing, cooking, baby care, sleeping, eating, ironing, cleaning, rest periods, breastfeeding, baby play—there is a never-ending list.

Keep your workload to a realistic time and expect no more than achieving a few items on your list. Your daily planner can keep you accountable.

Breastfeeding—is it fatiguing?
While it is a healthy choice to breastfeed your baby, you may feel fatigued, weary, and even sleepier than usual. The tip is not to get exhausted!

Pace yourself. The baby may want to cluster feed at times, and all you seem to be doing is feeding.

Days like this need you to power nap, and rest, leaving other chores un-ticked on your list or delegating to others.

High alert brain
As a result of the overwhelming sense of responsibility for a new baby and your recovery from major surgery, being on high brain alert is a behaviour we have often seen.

You will find yourself over-analysing, overreacting, and even losing your patience. Though quite reasonable, you can reset and reduce this high-alert sensation by taking 'time out' to rest, sleep, eat, and relax, perhaps with a warm bath.

Low blood sugar
Symptoms of low blood sugar can make you feel fatigued.

If you are not eating and drinking enough, this can lead to low blood sugar.

This is dangerous if you have had gestational diabetes or have Type 1 or Type 2 diabetes.

Energy comes from food and rest—do not complicate your recovery by not eating and drinking well.

Summary

With your new baby and recovering from a C-section wound, the likelihood of waking up tired and spending most of your early days postpartum longing for the chance of a whole night's sleep is inevitable. Our top tip is to power nap.

A useful website to check out is ICON resources—a great way to give ideas on coping with crying advice, and parents have found it very helpful: <https://iconcope.org/>.

Your body and your recovery will require many new experiences to be explored and lived. Sleep deprivation is inevitable at times, as your baby will need twenty-four-hour care and they have no idea of time or day. With good support networks around you, you can rescue some periods for your own sleep. As the body recovers from major surgery, you will most likely feel tired as the body is healing. The action hormone prolactin released during breastfeeding can also add to your tiredness.

A door note saying *sleeping new parents* is a great way to create space to power nap without being disturbed by visitors.

The essential factor is not to let fatigue overshadow your confidence and ability to learn and finally master some of the frustrations caused by lack of sleep. Looking sad and feeling sad is unpleasant. Learn to monitor yourself, and if the challenges you are feeling are affecting how you calm and enjoy your baby, do not blame yourself—admit it, and make sure you get help with it. There will always be a willing pair of helping hands to support you, and remember—looking after *you* means you can then look after your baby.

References

42. Five Guide—youtu.be/EwbLFdjHH_0

43. https://www.nhs.uk/conditions/pregnancy-and-baby/sleep-and-tiredness/

44. Stop That Shake- Babies Break—https://www.youtube.com/watch?v=TMyCrKPa6GI

45. Sudden Infant Death Syndrome—https://www.lullabytrust.org.uk/safer-sleep-advice/co-sleeping/

46. Postpartum Insomnia—https://www.mother.ly/life/postpartum-insomnia-is-realand-heres-what-you-can-do-about-it

47. The 1001 Critical Days-conception to two https://www.nspcc.org.uk/globalassets/documents/news/critical-days-manifesto.pdf https://iconcope.org/

Chapter 8
What do I need to know about my scar?

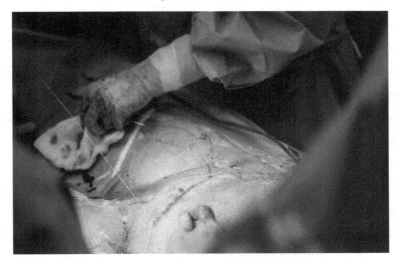

Why is it essential to read this chapter?

- To identify how your mindset can impact your pain and recovery.
- To feel well informed about the healing process and scar massage.
- To know how to clean, dress, and protect your wound.
- To understand preventative measures to avoid complications.
- To know signs of problems to look for and then to seek medical attention.
- To understand the importance of wound support and not straining.

For many women who have caesarean births, the scar is looked on as a symbol of life, hope bravery, and love. For other women, the scar can be a symbol of disappointment, shame, failure—even a source of anger and resentment, and some women cannot bear to even look at the scar. Coming home from hospital with a raw and painful incision is not easy, especially coupled with the 24/7 demands of your beautiful new baby. Healing takes time, and you can't push the process, but you can enhance the healing environment.

Although the C-section procedure is now considered routine, complications can include bleeding, infection, bladder injury, thromboembolic disease, foetal lacerations, admissions to high dependency units, and death. The rate of wound infections following a C-section range from 3–15% according to a 2020 Wounds International study.[48]

Understanding wound care and preventing complications is an essential part you can play in your recovery. Knowing what looks normal and abnormal along with what feels wrong can help you manage your wound recovery. Only you can rate your specific pain, soreness, and feeling unwell. How you deal with it can be the difference between wound infection and a more significant problem like sepsis.

Given that 3–15% of women will develop an infection in the postpartum period following C-section, viewing the video <https://youtu.be/gd1GVGvKolA> is encouraged so you know what to do and who to tell. The video explains the C-section healing process. This second video is a link about postpartum wound healing and the prevention of severe complications like sepsis: <https://youtu.be/cphHeFQvVxY>. Five Guide—Enhancing Awareness of Postpartum Sepsis. It does have a thought-provoking opening statement.

How do we heal?
Healing occurs in stages, and there are four processes involved: haemostasis, inflammatory, proliferative, and finally the maturation phase.[49] Haemostasis is the body's process that causes bleeding to stop. In most wounds, haemostasis will be spontaneous, but if there is excessive bleeding into the abdominal cavity, a wound drain tube will be temporarily in place to draw out any excess blood loss. A wound drain tube consists of a thin silicone tube with fine holes in the very end. It is inserted into the abdominal cavity at the time of surgery if required and stitched at skin level.

The tube allows for the drainage of fluid and gas from the body cavity after surgery. The amount and type of drainage from a drain is measured regularly. If you have a drain, it should be removed before leaving the hospital. This may be an uncomfortable experience, as the tube is often 120 centimetres long internally. The drain tube is sewn in place so pain relief will be important before removal. Sometimes tugging is necessary to remove the drain tube. Be sure to have pain medication before the removal.

A dressing will cover the small insertion hole. Remember this is an additional wound to heal, together with any other wounds or bruising from needle sites and intravenous drip sites or vaginal labouring wounds you may have experienced prior to an emergency C-section.

Scar types
T-scar/classical scar/bikini line.

Mothers who have a 'T' or 'J'-shaped uterine scar as opposed to a classical vertical incision are at higher risk for uterine rupture in future pregnancies. Be sure to ask your care team what type of scar you have. T-scars and laparotomy (horizontal) scars are usually associated with an emergency caesarean.

Figure 8.1 Five Guide logo

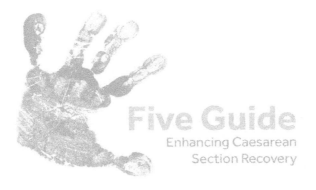

Challenges that can interrupt the healing process

As most surgical wound complications occur after discharge from the hospital, women and their partners can play a big role in early detection and intervention from healthcare professionals.

Some of the surgical wound complications are:

- Surgical site infection (SSI).
- Surgical wound dehiscence (SWD) or breakdown.
- Hyper-granulation, where the scar is raised above the skin surface.
- Peri-wound maceration—the skin becomes irritated and very red from the leakage.
- Medical adhesive-related skin injury (MARS).

Daily inspection and tracking of your wound are vital. You can use the scar tracker in Appendix 3 (Part Three) as a guide.

It is estimated that 2–8% of women will experience wound separation or breakdown, and 3–15% of women experience wound infections after caesarean section births. Undetected and untreated infections can lead to sepsis and, in extreme cases, death. Prevention of complications is the primary goal of managing your wound. Daily monitoring with a hand-held mirror looking for warning signs will help you catch any issues early. Using your scar tracker descriptions of abnormal signs will help you pick up early warning signs.

An SSI, as defined by the Centres for Disease Control (CDC), is an infection that presents up to thirty days after a surgical procedure and can appear at different times.

- 55% of SSIs are detected within 10 days of caesarean birth
- 75% of SSIs are detected within 14 days
- 90% of SSIs are detected within 20 days.[49]

my scar?

Abnormal signs & symptoms requiring medical review
- Fever
- Delay in your healing; gaping areas varying from pinprick size to larger openings
- Pus, redness, and pain getting worse
- Tenderness, warmth, and swelling near your wound
- Darkening skin at the edges
- Unpleasant odour.

How do I protect my scar from complications?
Key preventive measures for complications:

- Close monitoring for signs of SSI, SWD & sepsis using your scar tracker (Appendix 1)
- Reduce mechanical stress—use a splint, cushion, or rolled towel for wound support
- Reduce tension on suture line e.g., cryotherapy (ice packs) to reduce swelling
- Wound support e.g., elastic compression binder or wound splint to optimize pain relief
- Balanced nutrition and hydration
- Preventative antibiotics
- Clean wound environment
- Scar massage—to encourage blood to the area and soften the area
- Manage co-existing health conditions, e.g. diabetes
- Manage temperature post-surgery within normal range
- Clean wound dressings
- Daily self-assessment for any signs of abnormality
- Empty bladder and bowels regularly to avoid internal pressure on the stitches.

Your caesarean incision is your lasting reminder of the major surgery you underwent to deliver your baby. It will take six weeks for the five layers of stitches to heal fully in the absence of any complications.

The healing process begins as soon as the five layers are reunited and the skin closed with stitches, staples, or surgical glue.

Think about the Five Guide healing and five layers healing independent of one another—it will give you a visual picture of your anatomy and how much needs to heal and repair.

Specific wound care

Good wound hygiene is vital to help avoid infection: daily washing and careful pat drying with a clean towel used only for the wound. If more comfortable, place a sterile dressing over the wound inside your (preferably cotton) underwear.

Exudate is a pale coloured liquid produced by the body in response to tissue trauma. Some wounds produce more than others and the wound or scar becomes wet as the exudate leaks out. This exudate can cause excoriation of the skin close to the scar, so it is important to remove soggy dressings and keep the area as dry as possible. If the wound becomes too wet, it could also break down or split open.

Avoid tight clothing, wear loose outfits, and try to avoid squeezing into your old jeans, too.

This stage of recovery is one you really have some control over. You will be the first to see, feel, and experience the issues that may be symptomatic of a wound infection.

Wound dressings

Sterile absorbent dressings should always be used to cover the oozing wound. *Do not* put sanitary napkins on the wound; these are not sterile and may introduce infection.

Some doctors prefer negative pressure wound dressings that draw the exudate away from the scar, some of which operate with a pump attachment.

Be sure the tape used to hold the dressings isn't irritating your skin and causing trauma.

If you're concerned, closely observe the wound—using the scar tracker checklist—and seek medical advice if indicated.

To prevent overuse of antibiotics all other wound care hygiene measures should be observed, including nutrition, no smoking, and cleanliness. Antibiotics should only be prescribed if needed.

Many doctors are now using absorbent dressings which are interactive and attract bacteria and fungi away from the wound. These dressings are breathable and showerproof and also ensure protection against irritation from underwear and clothing.

Negative pressure wound therapy (NPWT) is sometimes used, whereby a special dressing (bandage) is sealed over the wound and a gentle vacuum pump is attached to draw out fluid and infection from the wound.

Wound splint
Using a C-section splint in your early days after surgery will aid and support your wound during the healing process.

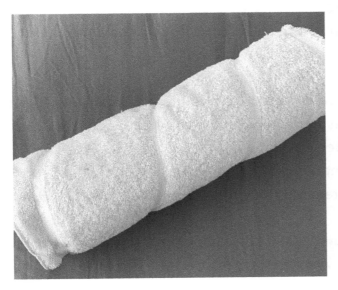

Any sudden movement—such as coughing, sneezing, or laughing, as well as heavy lifting—will raise the intra-abdominal pressure and cause strain on the internal stitches. This is known as mechanical stress and can cause stitches to burst open. Supporting the wound by gently holding a cushion, rolled up towel, or Caesarcare's surgical after care (SAC) splint during movement can help keep the wound stable, protecting it by reducing the impact of the sudden movement and possibly lowering the intrabdominal pressure on the healing layers. Splinting the wound can also increase your confidence to mobilise more easily.

We would be irresponsible as professionals if you were not informed about the dangers that can happen in your postpartum recovery. Wounds tell us a story—a story of good healing or delayed healing from complications. It is vital that wound management and care continues at home well beyond hospital discharge.

What to wear after a C-section?

Choose your comfy and cute post-C-section attire without any elastic waistbands. Over-the-bump attire like leggings, dungarees, and tunic-style outfits will stop any irritation on your wound. Shower, wear clean attire every day, and if you have a pendulous abdomen or tummy hangover, wear big cotton underwear that goes over the bump/scar. The bigger the knickers, the better it will feel, while they might not be your sexiest of underwear. The bigger underwear will facilitate wearing a sanitary pad. Internal sanitary products are not recommended during postpartum recovery period. Choose cotton fibre for its breathability; it will also be easier to wash and is less irritating on your skin.

A clean wound—key to good healing

Wound cleansing is essential to help reduce the infection risk and promote healing. There are five aspects of wound cleaning and care:

1. Before surgery—the incision area will need to have the pubic hair clipped or waxed, not shaved as that poses a risk from cuts. It will then be cleansed with surgical wash and draped with sterile cloth.
2. Avoid getting alcohol or detergents inside/onto the wound.
3. Decontaminate the wound by removing soiled dressings and reapplying clean dressings.
4. Clean the wound with warm water and pat dry with a clean cotton towel, used only once and exclusively for the wound.
5. Antibiotics may be prescribed for high-risk wounds or signs of infection.

Surgical site infection (SSI)

Surgical site infections (SSI's) occur when a wound becomes contaminated by bacteria, producing pain, redness, swelling, and potentially septic disease.[49] It is important to understand the healing process and the conditions that promote good healing. The stages of wound healing usually proceed in an organised way and follow four distinct processes. As most surgical wound complications occur after discharge from the hospital, you and your partner can play a big role in early detection and treatment from your healthcare provider.

The scar tracker located in the appendices will help with monitoring signs and symptoms of complications and when to consult your healthcare provider.

It is important to self-monitor your wound healing, as well as have your wound inspected by your home visiting maternity healthcare team, especially if you have diabetes or a high BMI. This inspection by a visiting HCP may not be a routine practice in all countries and states so it is important to be proactive in asking for an assessment.

Treatment

It is vital that you take ownership to follow the recommendations below.

- Take prescribed antibiotics.
- Wear clean clothes, wash/shower daily.
- Avoid putting sanitary pads over the wound.
- Show the healthcare team your wound, especially if you are concerned.
- Eat well and maintain nourishing healthy food and fluids; avoid smoking and alcohol, as these impede good tissue healing.

What is sepsis/postpartum sepsis?

Sepsis is a serious condition; do not ignore the symptoms.

Sepsis is an acute condition caused by your body's immune system responding abnormally to an infection, which can lead to tissue damage, organ failure, and death. Sepsis can occur in the days and weeks following C-section. The infection can happen in response to any injury or infection anywhere in the body[50] and can result from the following:

- a chest infection causing pneumonia
- a urine infection in the bladder
- a problem in the abdomen, such as a burst ulcer or a hole in the bowel
- an infected cut or bite
- a wound from trauma or surgery
- a leg ulcer or cellulitis.

Sepsis can be caused by a huge variety of different germs, like *Streptococcus*, *E. coli*, MRSA or *C. difficile*. Most cases are caused by common bacteria, which normally don't make us ill.[51]

How do I know if I might have sepsis?
You may feel like you have flu, gastroenteritis, or a chest infection at first. Early symptoms include fever, chills and shivering, a fast heartbeat, and quick breathing. Symptoms of sepsis or septic shock include feeling dizzy or faint, confusion or disorientation, nausea and vomiting, diarrhoea and cold, clammy and pale or mottled skin.

Sadly, sepsis is a life-threatening infection. If you feel unwell, tell someone.

If you feel you are getting worse, tell someone. Acting quickly and remembering that you are in the risk category for infection should make you and your support network more diligent in observing you.

Red Flag sepsis awareness tool
The United Kingdom Sepsis Trust has developed this source for health professionals to use in community practice. UK Sepsis Trust is a leading charity helping to save lives and improve education and outcomes for survivors. They raise public awareness, educate

health professionals, and support those affected by sepsis. If you present with any symptoms, seek help immediately![52]

Community educational resources are available at <https://www.global-sepsis-alliance.org/sepsis>.

Surgical wound dehiscence (SWD) or wound breakdown
Surgical dehiscence is a complication where the edges of a wound no longer meet or adhere together. Risks of this happening can lead to acute wound infection and wound breakdown. If you suspect this and see an opening in your wound, consult your healthcare practitioner. Separation may occur in one or several places and range from pinprick size to larger sections. Open wounds will need to be seen and dressed by your health care professional.

Risks factors for wounds that break down include
- Women with diabetes
- A large amount of wound exudate
- Not enough rest
- Lifting heavy objects
- A pre-existing wound abscess or blood clot
- Obesity and large BMI's
- Multiple C-sections.[53]

Figure 8.2 Wound breakdown
https://www.medicalnewstoday.com/articles/324505#pictures

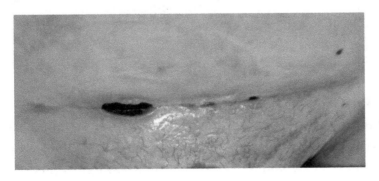

Bruising

Bruises are dark patches that appear under the skin surface where blood vessels have broken or burst and bled into tissues below. The colour can vary from red/blue to purple/yellow and even black. Bruises develop where there has been trauma.

It is common to see skin injury trauma after C-section. The darker the bruise, the more injury has occurred. Cold compresses help reduce bruising.

Bruises will naturally fade over days and weeks. It is important to remember the bruises you can see are likely to be deeper internally, hence the pain and discomfort.

A very gentle massage of the site will help break down the bruise, and will also aid capillary dilation and aid cell regeneration. Do not use any products on your skin at this stage. Remember visible bruising is an indicator for taking this recovery journey seriously.

Figure 8.3 post-surgery bruising

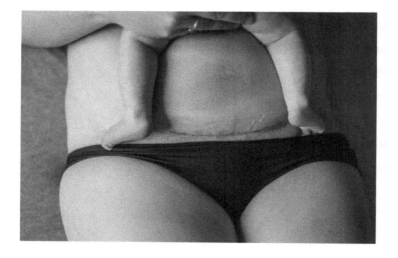

Psychological stress can affect healing

Stressors like pain, infection, fatigue, and inadequate nourishment are likely to cause psychological stress and impact the progress of wound healing. Seeking help from a postpartum therapist to reduce stress will be essential to enable your recovery.

Be kind to yourself; remind yourself that you have just had a baby and experienced major surgery. Taking time to recover your body will not let you 'rush it'.

Poor diet can affect healing

Nutrition—what you eat and when you eat—can affect how fast your body repairs. Nutrition and healing are intrinsically linked; specific nutrients in food are rich in minerals which aid tissue healing. Women with a high body mass index (BMI) are more prone to infection. So, attention to wound hygiene and monitoring is vital.

Without good nourishment, your body will struggle to heal, and your added fatigue of lack of sleep may lead to you becoming weak, which will in turn affect your wound-healing qualities. Poor nourishment does not provide your body with the minerals to heal.

Anaemia affects healing: iron or haemoglobin in the blood is responsible for blood oxygen and nutrient levels. So, any low haemoglobin level can inhibit wound healing. If you have had a substantial blood loss (over 500 mL) then you are likely to suffer from anaemia. Anaemia can cause some undesirable symptoms, like breathlessness, headaches, fainting, loss of appetite, metallic taste in your mouth, pale skin, and palpitations. If you experience any of the above symptoms, you should inform your health team. Blood transfusions can be essential if women have substantial blood loss volumes. Once the reason you have anaemia has been diagnosed (for example, blood loss during birth), your doctor will prescribe treatment. If your blood test shows your red blood cell count is low (deficient), you'll be prescribed iron tablets to replace the iron that's missing from your body. The prescribed tablets are more reliable than the supplements you can buy in pharmacies and supermarkets. You'll have to take them for about one month. Drinking orange juice at the time of ingestion may help your body absorb the iron. Some people get side effects like:

- constipation or diarrhoea
- tummy pain
- heartburn

- feeling sick
- black poop
- tasteless food.

Try taking the tablets with or soon after a meal to reduce the chance of side effects.

It's important to keep taking the tablets, even if you get side effects.

A wound abscess

Abscesses usually present as red, stiff, swollen, painful, fluid-filled raised bumps on your wound. They may be warm to the touch and may leak. They can develop internally or on the surface of your skin.

They might drain naturally or become so painful that they need surgical removal.

Most likely, they are because of a bacterial infection that will require antibiotics.

Due to the tenderness of the abscess, there will be pain, and analgesia should be taken. If you suspect an abscess is forming, seek medical advice quickly.

A wound blood clot or haematoma

A mass of blood tissue can form a clot. It can develop just under the skin surface; it happens as blood fibrins form together to stop bleeding. Blood that would typically escape before suturing does not run from the body—resulting in a blood clot.

Applying a cold compress should allow the vessels to constrict and stop blood loss.

However, blood clots on the suture line of your C-section should be handled gently, as the wound is more likely to break down. Eventually, as the process of cell, skin, and wound regeneration occurs, the clot should be absorbed naturally by the body.

Five layers of healing

As described in Chapter 2, there are five layers of tissue healing in progress. This healing process is explained in the Five Guide video, this set of pictures will help to visualise the healing from outside skin to internal womb.

1. Skin
2. Fat Layer
3. Muscle layer
4. Peritoneal Layer
5. Uterus

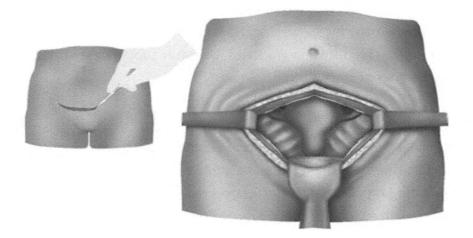

Figure 8.4 Five Guide Logo

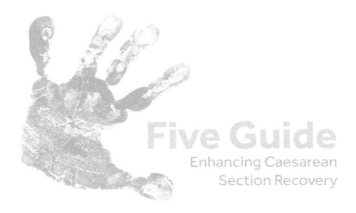

The five layers all need to heal and reshape and repair independently.[54]

Adhesions

Abdominal adhesions are bands of scar tissue. They can build up after any abdominal surgery, including C-section. The adhesions, which can cause concern and pain, are the connective tissue adhesions that form between organs like the bladder and the uterus. Preventing adhesions is part of the wound care regime of rest, recovery, proper nutrition, and emptying your bladder and bowels. It is challenging to prevent this from developing, and you would not know if it had developed until your next surgical procedure. Pain is usually an indicator of adhesions. Scar massage after the initial healing can support healthy internal tissue. Avoid lifting anything heavier than the weight of your new baby for six weeks. Straining muscles is easy if you are vacuuming floors and lifting wet laundry and groceries. Use your support network to help you or choose only to attempt small tasks.

Dressings/clips/wound closure strips

Caring for your wound will depend on what method of wound closure was used by your doctor. There is usually little choice as the surgeon and obstetric team will choose depending on availability and wound requirements. However, following new wound care guidance, and after much recent research into wound dehiscence, there are now available to surgical teams more wound-specific dressings—real alternative dressings to standard C-section wound care, helping to reduce the complications that may impede bonding or wound healing for new mothers. These absorbable and time usage dressings are of particular choice for women with large BMI or they have other complications like diabetes.

Surgical clips

Often made of stainless steel and used to staple/clip a wound together. They will need to be removed by a nurse using a specially designed clip remover between seven and ten days postoperatively.

Surgical beaded suture

A continuous suture beaded at two ends; this applies tension to the wound. It will need to be removed by a nurse between seven and ten days postoperatively.

Wound closure strips

Small, white, adhesive dressings. These will need to be removed by a nurse between seven to ten days postoperatively. This type of dressing can be secondary to another, like absorbable stitches. They can be used to secure a wound that might appear to be slightly opening.

Absorbable continuous suture line

This will be absorbed by the body and does not require removal. It will take up to twenty days for absorption to complete.

Surgeons will choose a method to suit the patient's size and wellbeing.

Knowledge is power; it will support your recovery if you know what is happening to you. Acting on anything you are not happy with is vital. Your body, your recovery!

How long will it take for my C-section wound to heal?

If you have no complications during or after your C-section, then wound healing will be between five and six weeks for initial recovery. Accomplishing complete healing will depend on many of the things we have discussed: rest, wound hygiene, wound assessment, pain relief, cleanliness, rest, and recovery. The complete healing will take up to one year. We ask you to think at six weeks, *Should I return to exercise and all the duties and activities I did before birth?* Your body will set the pace; the pain and the fatigue you will experience will be indicators that you are overdoing it. Many HCPs advise not to get pregnant for up to a year after a C-section in order to allow the internal scars to heal; remember, there are five of them! Contraception is a serious conversation you should be having if you have a C-section. Scars need to heal before they can be stretched again.

Take a wound photo regularly

Taking a photo of your wound provides both a clinical history review on the healing progress and a reminder of what you endured. It can also be used to show a doctor what your concern is. Taking regular photos provides a history of your recovery. Any new symptoms, as you can see in the images we have chosen, are a reflection of wound care and recovery. Keep a photo diary of your wound healing as it has many uses:

- treatment options
- signs and symptoms of healthy or compromised recovery
- reflection
- recovery
- acceptance
- body image changes.

When to use scar-healing products

There are many products to support scar healing, including gels, oils, and creams, but none should be used until there is complete skin closure and healing. This will take up to six weeks if there have been no complications. Scarring is part of the course of the surgery; the skin will start to heal, and it will be up to you to support that healing process. Everyone has a different healing rate. We have discussed what will promote your healing. Do not use anything that will cause inflammation or a chemical-based product that could affect the normal healing process. Scars are an unavoidable part of your birth; accepting your birth scar with confidence is the focus. It will take up to a year for you to see just what scarring is left.

What about scar massage?

Some healthcare professionals, such as physiotherapists and occupational therapists, offer scar massage, and it may be something you may find helpful after six weeks. Prior to six weeks, the area can be massaged through intentional deep belly breathing mobilising the internal tissues.

Caesarean birth can sometimes be a traumatic experience, depending on the circumstances. Massaging the C-section scar can help you work through difficult emotions and is therapeutic beyond the physical needs.

Studies show soft tissue mobilisation techniques (massage) have excellent benefits, including:[55]

- desensitising the area.
- reducing pain
- reducing adhesions and scar tissue
- allowing touch and acceptance of the scar
- lessening the development of keloid scar tissue
- stimulating vascular activity to the area.

Scar area numbness after C-section
It is common to find the area around your scar numb after a C-section at first but, over time, the nerve sensation will return.

Vaginal trauma included?
Vaginal trauma may also have been experienced and healing will be included in your recovery, especially if you had tried to deliver vaginally. Injury can often consist of bruising and tearing or cutting in the event of an episiotomy. Vaginal soreness and trauma may also have needed suturing. You must keep the pubic area clean and dry. When on the toilet, vaginal hygiene can be enhanced with a simple jug of warm water poured through your legs onto your perineum into the toilet as you urinate or poo. This is kind to a sore perineum and eases haemorrhoids or washes away blood loss easily. Pat dry and keep clean at each toilet visit.

Bleeding that is not associated with uterine healing can complicate your recovery. Be aware of your birthing journey if you tried to deliver and the birth plan proceeded to an emergency C-section.[56] Be mindful that you may have more to heal than you thought.

Figure 8.5 Wound care

Wound Care Principles

Cleaning and Dressing

- Dressing left intact for 48 hrs post-surgery or as per manufacturer instructions.
- Wash hands before dressing.
- Use new, clean dressings.
- Dispose of used dressings in a sealed bag.
- Timely changing of dressings to avoid wound damage.
- Avoid pressure from underwear or clothing.

Environment

- Maintain normal body temperature.
- Splint wound to reduce mechanical stress.
- Expose to fresh air for a short after the shower.
- Avoid smoking.
- Avoid contamination from foreign bodies, e.g. dust from hairdryers.
- Manage pre-existing conditions, e.g. diabetes.
- Avoid strenuous activity.

Nutrition and Medication

- Some medications, for example steroids, can delay healing.
- Nutritional deficiencies can delay the healing rate.
- Include foods rich in protein Vitamins A, C and E, and minerals such as zinc, and magnesium.
- Intake 1.5—2 litres of water daily.
- Take regular pain relief to facilitate gentle exercise.
- Iron deficiencies can also delay healing.

Self-inspection

- Daily self-inspection of the scar with a wall mirror or handheld mirror.
- Take a healing photo log. Any deviation from normal, show your health care professional.
- Ask for help if necessary.
- Use a scar tracking document to note any deviations from normal, i.e, swelling, odour, gaping, increased pain, or redness.

McKnight Cowan. J & Rastas, LM. (2022)

Summary

Many of the thousands of women we have cared for have had issues with their caesarean scar. We have come to learn and understand the profound effect that C-section birth can have on both physical and mental health. The surgical scar can evoke many different feelings, many of which are not spoken about. There may be fear and anxiety about touching your tummy or looking at your abdomen or scar. These common feelings can be associated with the pain, guilt or shame, pride, or regret, to name a few. It can be helpful to share your feelings with a trusted person and to get help to process them if necessary. Your emotions relating to recovery will be individual to you. It is different for everyone, but we have also come to know that no two C-section recovery journeys will be the same. Try to look at your scar and think about it; why don't you write in your journal what that scar means to you? Photograph it and use the snaps as a recovery journey or learn to recover your emotional connection on the wound that gave a 'door to life'.

Be mindful of what you see and how you react. Wound infections can appear very quickly after surgery and up to thirty days postoperatively. Do not ignore any signs and symptoms that give pain or alarm you.

Rest and mindful self-compassion, combined with a nutritious diet, will enhance the healing process. Listen to your body and let it help you set the pace for recovery.

Keep your scar clean, keep it dry, let the healing process begin; it is a long process involving many anatomical layers. Each layer is independent of the other, and each layer will have different periods of recovery time.

Over to you. Remember: to heal well is to care well for yourself.

—Janine

References

48. Sandy-Hodgetts K et al (2020) International best practice recommendations for the early identification and prevention of surgical wound complications. Wounds International

49. World Union of Wound Healing Societies (WUWHS) Consensus Document. Surgical wound dehiscence: improving prevention and outcomes. Wounds International, 2018

50. https://www.sepsis.org/sepsisand/pregnancy-childbirth/

51. Sepsis Alliance (2020) Pregnancy, Childbirth & Sepsis retrieved from https://www.sepsis.org/education/resources/posters-and-infographics/

52. Red Flag Sepsis Awareness. https://sepsistrust.org/wp-content/uploads/2018/06/GP-adult-NICE-Final-2.pdf

53. https://www.sepsis.org/sepsis-basics/symptoms/

54. https://www.britishskinfoundation.org.uk/blog/the-benefits-of-scar-massage

55. Pelvic floor disorders—https://www.ncbi.nlm.nih.gov/pmc/articles/PMC3681820/

56. https://rcni.com/primary-health-care/features/simple-visual-tool-helps-safeguard-mothers-after-caesarean-section-150506

Chapter 9
Maternal mental health—how am I supposed to feel?

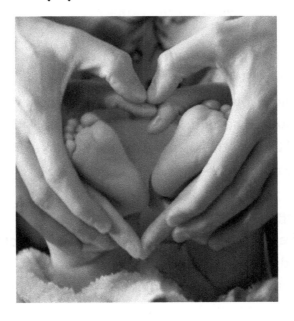

Why should I read this chapter?

- To realise you are not alone.
- To identify negative emotions, and when to seek help.
- To understand the importance of journaling and sharing your journey.
- To learn how to ask for help.

Understanding your headspace after birth

The transition to motherhood can be overwhelming and, at times, you may feel like your brain function has altered. This is nature's way of keeping you focused on you and your baby's needs, and in time, you will regain mental clarity.

The postpartum period is a time to understand what your mental health endures following pregnancy and birth surgery. It is normal for emotional changes during the transition to your new role of motherhood.

It is very common to experience mixed emotions after surgical birth: on the one hand, you are over the moon about your beautiful baby's arrival, on the other hand, you are feeling low in energy and troubled by pain and discomfort expected after major surgery. As discussed in the debrief earlier in Chapter 3, the intensity of feelings will directly relate to the circumstances before surgery.

If you feel things are not quite right, there are two useful tools to assess your emotions— the Whooley Questions (Fig. 9.1) and Edinburgh scale (Fig. 9.2)—in this chapter summary, which will help you explore your feelings and identify whether further help from a health professional is needed. We explore them a little further into this chapter; we advise you to read through this chapter to gain insight into understanding why they are used and when to use them.

Sharing your feelings and emotions

Midwife Laura Godfrey-Isaacs recommends journaling for mothers to help restore some balance around the new feelings and challenges they may experience both physically and emotionally. She has teamed with creative individuals to create free resources to help mothers set up their maternal journal groups.[57]

Journaling can also be a helpful way of tracking your progress and identifying early warning signs. This manual includes the rationale and a variety of suggestions for methods of recording your postpartum journey.

'Baby brain' or 'mental fog' is real, with neuroscience explaining it and how it changes motherhood brains. You will also learn about the benefits of the baby brain and how to use strategies for raising and lowering the baby brain phenomenon.[58]

Why, how, what can I be feeling?

The following paragraphs will explore a variety of postnatal mental health issues. Exploring these feelings and emotions will help you to understand the why element of how they affect you, and what you can do to help yourself.

Anxiety after a C-section

Anxiety can occur as a response after surgical birth and especially after a traumatic birth. Many women can feel tearful, unable to cope, and reflect on the birth with anxiety and upset. There is a rapid change after birth in your hormone levels that regulate emotions. So, your emotions can lead to anxieties that bring mixed mood swings, often called 'the blues'. Hopefully, this won't last longer than two weeks. Tell your partner and your healthcare professional how you feel. Do not bottle up the feelings that cause you anxiety.

Depression before/after C-section

'Baby blues' and postpartum depression include symptoms of mood swings and emotional states of change. If you have suffered from depression antenatally, then it is more likely you could feel depression returning after birth. You are coping with these changes and experiences after C-section; it takes longer to recover compared to vaginal birth. Mental health awareness and care are essential. Reactions and adjustments you make to function must be a priority. Suggested reading: NHS depressed after birth resources.[59] Try to remember how you coped before baby. It is a sign of positive parenting and self-care if you ask for help or feel yourself 'falling' emotionally. We ask you not to set yourself up for a fall by doing too much; getting tired and fatigued will make depressive thoughts more. Be mindful of your own coping mechanisms.

Some Australian First Nations Women may experience anxiety and depression as a result of the trauma of having to leave your land and people and being denied your spiritual and cultural practices for birthing. Having a caesarean birth may cause you to feel shame and sorrow, as if you have done something culturally wrongly by not having your baby on country. The hospital environment can invoke feelings of fear and loneliness in contrast to the nurturing, private, and gentle practice of birthing on country whilst being supported by known and trusted women. It will be important to seek out an Indigenous health care provider or one who is familiar with First Nations peoples cultural birthing traditions who can help you debrief such an experience and support your healing and reconnection with the land and sacred traditions. It can be helpful to include your cultural practice wishes in your birth plan also. Other helpful services to help with your healing can be found in the following resources:

- Women's Business Manual <https://docs.remotephcmanuals.com.au/review/g/manuals2017-manuals/d/20293.html?publication=rphcm-001>.
- Gayaa Dhuwi (Proud Spirit) Australia <https://www.gayaadhuwi.org.au/if-you-need-help/>.
- Promoting Perinatal Mental Health Wellness in Aboriginal and Torres Strait Islander Communities <https://earlytraumagrief.anu.edu.au/files/chapter16.pdf>.

Crying and emotional upset after birth

With the baby blues, you may become sad and feel like crying at both happy and sad things. One minute you may be tearful, and the next happy. Feeling overwhelmed after birth is quite common. But, if it lasts more than ten days and you feel you are struggling, get yourself checked out or answer the Whooley Questions.[60]

The Whooley questions act as a short self-reflection of where you are and how you are feeling.

Fatigue

If you are very tired after birth, remember you are not alone. The causes of fatigue are further discussed and explored in the sleep chapter (Chapter 7).

A lot of things can make you tired and fatigued after birth; multitasking is probably one of the highest on the list. What you can do about it is further discussed in our sleep and coping chapter. For further information read the article titled '10 unexpected reasons new moms feel so tired—and what to do about it'.[61]

Postpartum depression

Approximately one in ten mothers can develop postpartum medical depression following birth.[62]

Support and understanding from family, friends, and sometimes from a professional such as a health visitor, GP, midwife, or psychologist can help you to recover. Other treatment options include psychological treatments, such as cognitive behavioural therapy or antidepressant medicines. Support groups and walking groups can also be very beneficial.

Talking to other women with a similar experience can help to 'normalise' your feelings and how you cope.

Find out what is available in your locality; community support groups provide invaluable support for new parents. You are not alone. There is always help available—just reach out. Do it for you, your baby, your family.

Mood swings that make you feel ill, low, and depressed must not be ignored; share your feelings with a trusted friend, partner, or health professional. It is important to clearly identify your feelings. Postnatal anger and rage can be scary and being told to 'Calm down' can lead to symptoms of unrelenting hostility.[63]

These symptoms pose a red-flag warning for some women who are experiencing such distress and anxiety post-birth.

Uncontrollable anger can be a symptom of postpartum depression, and you need support and assessment by a health professional. Be safe, be gentle with your baby, and get help. Accepting help is a strength, you can then get the right help and support you need so you can recover and be the momma you want to be.[64]

Screening for postpartum depression

Valuable screening tools are available to support assessment and treatment planning. Two we have used in our clinical practice are the Whooley Questions and the Edinburgh Postnatal Depression Scale. Both tools can explore behaviour associated with the risk of depression.

Undiagnosed postpartum depression is unacceptable in today's world—women can be supported. However, use of these tools without professional support is not recommended. If you feel you need help, it is a sign of good parenting and self-help to get it. More information can be found on the NHS website.

Antidepressant medication after birth

Depression levels can become high enough to require medication. However, there will be some medications that are not suitable after birth or while breastfeeding.

With appropriate treatment and support, women can make a full recovery.

Just like iron medication for iron deficiency anaemia can restore your blood levels to normal, antidepressant medication can restore mental health.

Be realistic about an assessment of your mental health, including if medication is required to support and aid your recovery.

Good nutrition, adequate fluids, and rest are also important to mental health and wellness.

Perinatal Anxiety & Depression Australia (PANDA) offer helpful resources in relation to rest, diet, and self-care.

Postpartum depression therapy

Speak to your medical team if you think you may have postpartum depression. There are various therapies to support you, not just medication.

There are several therapies to support your recovery; these include:

- self-help strategies
- group/individual therapies
- medication
- group events
- behavioural therapies
- hospitalisation
- journaling—write about your feelings.

Hormonal changes after birth commonly affect mental and physical wellbeing.

Postpartum depression is associated with many risk factors, both psychological and physiological, including fluctuations in hormone levels.

Many new mothers experience symptoms of irritability, low mood, and mental health compromise. But most can be related to hormonal changes and are often called 'the blues'.

Postpartum psychosis

This is a rare and severe mental health illness, characterised by sudden and dramatic changes in a woman's thinking, mood, and behaviour. It can affect a woman normally in the first four weeks but can occur up to twelve weeks. Previous mental health illnesses can make you more susceptible to this illness.[65]

Treatment, including medication and often hospitalisation, may be required. Specialist units provide mother and baby units. Read more on the NHS website. A strong supportive family/friend network is required if you are diagnosed with this condition.

Post-birth reflection/birth debrief

After a stressful or traumatic birth, women should be offered and advised to perform a birth debrief. Carefully considering the possibilities that birth reflection and birth can expose a condition like post-traumatic stress disorder (PTSD). PTSD will require professional help and support. Secrets to a positive debrief are:

- The timing of it.
- The person who is supporting the reflection.
- The offer of support following outcomes.
- Positive listening skills.
- Understanding and knowledge of events.
- Ability to support or refer the woman to enhanced services if required.

Chapter 3 of this manual outlines the birth debriefing process. A birth debrief questionnaire provides an opportunity to get answers to emotional concerns and stressors. A good birth debrief should be able to answer the *why*, *what*, and *how* events happened that may be the cause of any emotional anxieties you are experiencing. Informed and sensitive information on events may help you to understand and absorb what happened to you while giving birth. It may then be easier to accept and internalise emotionally what has given rise to heightened emotions.

Sadness, disappointment, anger, violation, loss of self-esteem, guilt, loss of control: these are all emotions that can cause varying degrees of emotional compromise after C-section. 'Guilt' is a word we learn as children, but defining it as a feeling or emotional state is less understood. What is specific about these words is the effect they have upon our beliefs and values of ourselves.

Remember, in the situation you found yourself in at the birth of your baby, you may not have had any control. So, reflect carefully, as you may not have the choices you would generally have had control over—choices and decisions made about you or your baby at the time of birth.

Relaxation to support postnatal mental health

Relaxation techniques reduce muscle tension. Relaxation exercises can help decrease the effects of stress on your mind and body and spiritual wellbeing. Some relaxation techniques blend breathing, massage, meditation, music, and sleep. Practising relaxation techniques can have many benefits, including:

- Slowing heart rate and breathing rate.
- Lowering blood pressure.
- Improving digestion.
- Maintaining normal blood sugar levels.
- Reducing the activity of stress hormones, which reduces anger and frustration.
- Increasing blood flow to major muscles.
- Reducing muscle tension and chronic pain.
- Improving concentration and mood, which boosts confidence to handle problems.
- Improving sleep quality, which lowers fatigue.

Laughter is both medicinal and relaxing and can provide a great antidote to stress, so it's good to try to inject laughter into your day. There are many funny podcasts, TV shows, and movies that can transport you into laughter and release a good dose of endorphins. Don't take yourself too seriously; maybe call a friend who makes you laugh. It is a gift to be able to laugh your way out of stressful situations. Of course, have your wound splint or cushion at the ready to support your belly laughs.

Learning to laugh at yourself is an instrumental art also.

We are sure your new baby will make you laugh, especially if that new nappy is not on tight enough and you are blessed with a wet patch or deposit on your clothing.

Tokophobia

Tokophobia is a pathological fear of pregnancy and birth. It is rare, and symptoms can result in the request for an elective C-section.

Pregnancy and childbirth are significant events in many women's lives. While it can be a time of great joy, it can also be a source of stress and anxiety. Women often worry about the usual pain of childbirth and the possibility of something going wrong. These are all reasonable concerns that almost all pregnant women experience to some degree.

Requesting a C-section for fear of birth always, in our experience, finds women going through many hoops to discuss it with a surgeon and may result in you speaking with a psychiatric doctor as well.

Mother-child relationships—bonding and attachment concerns

Attachment is one specific aspect of the relationship between a parent and their baby. Feelings and actions provide the distinction between attachment and bonding.

Attachment is about both you and your baby. It's about how you build a relationship over time that helps your baby feel secure, loved, and ready to face the world.

Bonding is all about you. It's about the surge of love and tenderness you feel for your baby. You may feel it when you're pregnant, perhaps when you see the first blurry image of your baby in an ultrasound. Or you may feel it when you first hold your baby after giving birth, but it can take longer.

Attachment and bonding go hand in hand, though. It follows that if you feel a strong bond with your baby, your baby is more likely to develop a secure attachment to you.

Be aware attachment and bonding can be negatively affected by negative emotions such as shame, guilt, and disappointment or pain, so be sure to keep those in check.

Fear of future pregnancy/miscarriage

Becoming pregnant again after birth or miscarriage involves an emotional investment in planning, choice, and fear of loss.

Fear is associated with protective self-choices and protective abilities. Making the right choices about contraception, sexual relationships, and reproductive health are vital and need supportive services to address any fears you have.

Losing a pregnancy involves feelings of grief and loss and what some women describe as a feeling of 'empty arms'. Losing a baby and then delivering another baby can trigger memories and feelings of regret, sadness, and loss. Handling the associated anxiety of loss takes time for healing and can be terrifying. Losing a baby can impact your ability to enjoy the safe birth of another child.

Supportive maternity services are available and should be encouraged for any woman experiencing fear and loss after miscarriage.[66]

Hormonal changes and effects postnatally

Typically, expect to experience hormonal changes for the first six to eight weeks after birth. Menstrual periods may not return in a timely manner, and breastfeeding hormones and healing enzymes will all affect your neuroendocrinological wellbeing.

The imbalance is all a response to healing and recovery. Be sensitive to your estrogen and progesterone female hormone levels as they rise and fall in the postpartum recovery period.

The emotional highs and the lows need to be discussed as your body's hormones will play a part in your personality and behaviours.

Indigenous/cultural mothers experiences postpartum

Addressing postpartum depression and maternal mental health compromise in different cultural groups need careful service planning, and access to these services should be made available to all women.

Postpartum depression has profound effects on the quality of life, social functioning, and economic productivity of women and families; whatever culture you are from, do not suffer in silence and get help. Accepting help and support is the key as not all fixes can come from culture, religion, or alternative therapies.

Body image after birth

Body image after birth can affect how you perceive yourself—being brutally honest with yourself too early after birth can lead to anxiety.

Give yourself time to recover, adapt, and restore activities like exercise and controlled diet intake to support your return to a pre-birth figure.

It took forty weeks to grow a baby; it will take as long to restore your body to a pre-pregnant and acceptable state.

Social pressure is causing women to suffer body image issues.

Have discussions with your partner about this; encourage their support as you deal with new roles and emotional and physical changes and challenges.

Although healthy, some women will struggle with body image issues. Overcoming them could require therapy.[67] Being bigger, bumpy, or lumpy for a while postpartum is normal; after all, it took you nine months to grow a baby—it will take some months for your body to recover and reshape.

Guilt, disappointment after birth

While you might not have expected to feel guilty or disappointed, emotions experienced by women are unique.

Guilt and disappointment can present as gender disappointment, birth choices, mode of birth, injury, neonatal unit admissions. There are many presentations; coping with the emotional spin-off is the key to recovery.

Perspective and a positive birth debrief, and reflection is essential.

Further information about coping with emotions can be found on Tommy's website.[68] We again encourage you to journal your emotions—this will help to support you in identifying your concerns and timeline your feelings. It can also support you to reflect on how you have previously felt and allow you to see personal emotional change.

What is birth trauma?

Birth trauma is another name for post-traumatic stress disorder (PTSD) after birth.[69]

In the UK alone, an estimated 3–4% of mothers develop PTSD. Some partners suffer PTSD, too, from witnessing a traumatic birth. Getting support is the key to recovery. Things that can make a traumatic birth include: feelings of loss of control; feeling unsupported by staff, or that staff were hostile; lack of pain relief; frightening or distressing events that made the birth utterly different from what you expected; lengthy labour or short and very intense labour; induction; forceps or vacuum extraction birth; emergency C-section; loss of blood (haemorrhage); fear of death or permanent injury; birth of a baby who is injured or disabled or ill; stillbirth; your baby having to spend time in NNU; premature birth; maternal collapse; or general anaesthetic.

What are the symptoms of PTSD? You may experience:

- Reliving the worst parts of the birth over and over again, or flashbacks.
- Feeling jumpy and overanxious.
- Finding it difficult to bond with the baby.
- Having difficulty sleeping, insomnia.
- Experiencing memory of the birth inaccurately.
- Feeling depressed, irritable, and angry.
- Finding it difficult to concentrate.
- Finding it hard to breastfeed.
- Palpitations, sweating, panic attacks.

You may still feel traumatised even if experiencing only one or two of these symptoms.

Birth is completely unpredictable, so you should never feel guilty about traumatic birth, but PTSD can make you feel that way.

> **Leonie's PTSD story**
>
> My fifth caesarean was particularly traumatic as the spinal anaesthetic only partially blocked the sensation, so I was able to feel the cutting, pulling and pushing, and the stitching. I remember trying to kick the doctors but with no feeling in my legs, I had no option but to bear with the pain. The junior doctor wasn't prepared to do a general anaesthetic without a senior doctor. I managed to push through the excruciating pain by praying and going into a deep meditative state. The senior anaesthetist later apologised for the experience, and for three months, I got on with life with my new baby. Then one day I read an article by a woman who had surgery and had had a failed anaesthetic. She described the sensation as a hot knife slicing through butter. That was my trigger, the terror came flooding back, and I descended into PTSD. I became a hyper anxious, hyper vigilant, insomniac, and non-trusting of anaesthesia, to the point where my dentist could not deaden my gum despite many attempts. Finally, my local doctor recommended hypnosis to help erase the memory. After two sessions, I was ready to face the dentist again, and thankfully my gum was deadened after the first injection. PTSD is real and very debilitating, however, today it is more recognised and treatable. Don't suffer in silence; seek help is my advice.

Treatment for PTSD

Two main treatments are:

- Trauma-focused cognitive-behavioural therapy (CBT)

CBT can help you understand and process what you went through and change how you think about your experience, including finding ways to improve your state of mind.[70]

- Eye movement desensitisation and reprocessing (EMDR)

This is a technique that involves watching a moving object or listening to a series of taps through headphones. Although it sounds strange, the results are valid. It appears to be a way of stopping flashbacks and feelings by moving them into your long-term memory.

How to get help for PTSD
Referral through your doctor to see a therapist who specialises in PTSD.[71]

It may overwhelm you at first, but with help, support, and a network around you, coping and caring will come together, and the anxiety will cease.

Partner's emotional wellbeing after a birth
Becoming two parents will put a strain on both of you. Partners see but do not feel the pain of childbirth. For some partners, this can result in PTSD, anxiety, and depression. Partners, dads, and birth partners can all present with anxieties following a C-section, or vaginal birth. They, too, can get support, and in doing so they in turn can help you.

Any of the symptoms we have listed can affect your partner, so it is essential to be aware of what changes you, can also affect your partner. Discuss it and support them too.

Fear of death in childbirth
To be scared to die during childbirth is a genuine phenomenon.

Sometimes people, women, and their partners can't get over it without therapy. PTSD is an involuntary response to trauma, not something you choose. Symptoms and flashbacks result in anxiety and can affect your reproductive choices and wishes ahead.

People diagnosed with PTSD or symptoms of PTSD need to have their terror stopped. With the right treatment and support, women and their partners will recover to make informed future choices.

Whooley Questions for depression screening

These are simple and easy to use the questions designed to get you thinking about how you are feeling. A health professional may well ask you these questions. Be honest and realistic as you may need to be referred to other professionals for support.

Figure 9.1 Whooley scale[72]

Whooley Questions

1. During the past month, have you often been bothered by feeling down, depressed or hopeless? ☐ Yes ☐ No

2. During the past month, have you often been bothered by little interest or pleasure in doing things? ☐ Yes ☐ No

"Yes" to one (or both) questions = positive test(requires further evaluation)

"No" to both questions = negative test (depressed)

Test Characteristics | Whooley Questions
whooleyquestions.ucsf.edu

Scoring your emotional scale on the EPDS tool[73]

Scoring is better derived if done by a qualified health professional, especially as they can then develop a care plan for you that is tailored specifically for your needs.

- A score of more than 10 suggests minor or major depression may be present.
- Postpartum depression occurs after giving birth. Symptoms are present for most of the day and last for at least two weeks.

The EPDS tool can be used several times over different phases of a recovery.

Any tool is only as good as the user; identifying any emotional ill health will require a holistic collection of signs and symptoms, in order to prepare an effective recovery plan.

Responsibility means it is your job to protect, care for, and nurture the safety and wellbeing of your baby. Creating a state of anxiety and accountability of having to deal with this in addition to your recovery will increase any anxieties you had previously.

Perinatal mental health (PMH) problems are those that occur during pregnancy and can exist within the first year after a baby's birth. The physical and emotional and spiritual wellbeing of a new mother go hand in hand, each interlinking with wellbeing and recovery.

During pregnancy, childbirth, and mothering, there will be hormonal changes affecting thought and actions. The level of support and care a mother receives at that time will affect her outcomes and mental wellbeing. Quite honestly, in our experience, mothers tend to worry about housework and cleaning over and above rest and recuperation.

There has been a change in attitude toward maternal mental wellbeing in recent decades. It is now acknowledged as good practice to routinely ask about mental health. Questions about the mother's mental health are now asked throughout the course of pregnancy and postpartum recovery.

All women deserve to enjoy the gift of life and maternal wellbeing, whether their journey into motherhood was uneventful or traumatic. Every parent deserves to nurture a new life and enjoy his or her mental wellbeing, too.

In this chapter, we call out to all the women we have cared for who have suffered postpartum depression. We hope that you reading this chapter shows that your voice will be heard.

Let your questions and the answers we have highlighted reflect hidden voices and the struggles and paths some new mothers may take.

Tell someone; help someone to be the parent they want to be.

Families and carers play an invaluable role in helping mothers and their families to recover from perinatal mental health problems. Their contribution as partners in care must be recognised and valued and access support themselves as individuals in their caring role.

Figure 9.2 Edinburgh Post Natal Depression Scale
Edinburgh Postnatal Depression Scale (EPDS)

*Cox JL, Holden JM Sagovsky R (1987) Detection of postnatal depression: development of the 10-item Edinburgh postnatal depression scale. Brit J Psychiatry 150 782-86. Reproduced with permission.

Name:

Date:

We would like to know how you have been feeling in the past week. Please indicate which of the following comes closest to how you have been feeling over the past seven days, not just how you feel today. Please tick one circle for each question that comes closest to how you have felt in the last seven days.

Here is an example already completed.

Have felt happy:
1. Yes, all of the time
2. Yes, most of the time
3. No, not very often
4. No, not at all

This would mean: 'I have felt happy most of the time during the past week'. Please complete the other questions in the same way.

Maternal mental health—how am I supposed to feel?

1. I have been able to laugh and see the funny side of things.
    1. As much as I always could
    2. Not quite so much now
    3. Definitely not so much now
    4. Not at all

2. I have looked forward with enjoyment to things.
    1. As much as I ever did
    2. Rather less than I used to
    3. Definitely less than I used to
    4. Hardly at all

3. I have blamed myself unnecessarily when things went wrong.
    1. Yes, most of the time
    2. Yes, some of the time
    3. Not very often
    4. No, never

4. I have been anxious or worried for no good reason.
    1. No, not at all
    2. Hardly ever
    3. Yes, sometimes
    4. Yes, very often

5. I have felt scared or panicky for no very good reason.
    1. Yes, quite a lot
    2. Yes, sometimes
    3. No, not much
    4. No, not at all

6.   Things have been getting on top of me.
     1.   Yes, most of the time I haven't been able to cope at all
     2.   Yes, sometimes I haven't been coping as well as usual
     3.   No, most of the time I have coped quite well
     4.   No, I have been coping as well as ever

7.   I have been so unhappy that I have had difficulty sleeping.
     1.   Yes, most of the time
     2.   Yes, sometimes
     3.   Not very often
     4.   No, not at all

8.   I have felt sad or miserable.
     1.   Yes, most of the time
     2.   Yes, quite often
     3.   Not very often
     4.   No, not at all

9.   I have been so unhappy that I have been crying.
     1.   Yes, most of the time
     2.   Yes, quite often
     3.   Only occasionally
     4.   No, never

5.   The thought of harming myself has occurred to me.
     1.   Yes, quite often
     2.   Sometimes
     3.   Hardly ever
     4.   Never

Summary

An overwhelming sense of responsibility after birth is experienced by many new parents. There is now not only you to be responsible for.

While there was previously only you to worry about, motherhood brings with it the added anxiety and responsibility of care and attention of a vulnerable newborn baby.

References

57. https://www.maternaljournal.org/what-is-maternal-journal

58. Baby Brain phenomena- retrieved from—https://neurosciencenews.com/mommy-brain-attention-16573/

59. Feeling Depressed after birth retrieved from https://www.nhs.uk/conditions/pregnancy-and-baby/feeling-depressed-after-birth/

60. Whooley Questionnaire Retrieved from https://www.nationalelfservice.net/mental-health/depression/whooley-questions-have-high-sensitivity-and-modest-specificity-in-the-detection-of-depression/

61. https://www.mother.ly/life/10-unexpected-reasons-new-moms-feel-so-tiredand-what-to-do-about-it

62. https://www.nhs.uk/conditions/pregnancy-and-baby/mental-health-problems-pregnant/

63. Postnatal Anger. Retrieved from https://www.nhs.uk/conditions/pregnancy-and-baby/feeling-depressed-after-birth/PostnatalAnger

64. Uncontrollable anger. Retrieved from https://postpartumprogress.com/uncontrollable-anger-can-be-part-of-postpartum-depression

65. NHS Postpartum Psychosis. Retrieved from https://www.nhs.uk/conditions/post-partum-psychosis/Fatigue postpartum

66. Miscarriage .retrieved from https://www.nhs.uk/conditions/miscarriage/afterwards/

67. https://undefiningmotherhood.com/postpartum-body-image/

68. Coping with emotions after C-section—https://www.tommys.org/pregnancy-information/labour-birth/caesarean-section/coping-emotions-after-c-section

69. PTSD retrieved from https://www.nct.org.uk/labour-birth/you-after-birth/traumatic-birth-and-post-traumatic-stress-disorder

70. CBT for postnatal depression -retrieved from https://www.mindbody7.com/news/2019/4/25/treating-postpartum-depression-with-cognitive-behavioral-therapy

71. Getting Help for PTSD visit or www.birthtraumaassociation.org.uk

72. Whooly,A.(N.D) Whooley questions for Depression Screening. Retrieved from https://whooleyquestions.ucsf.edu/

73. Edinburgh Post Natal Depression Scale retrieved from https://www.cope.org.au/wp-content/uploads/2018/02/EPDS-Questionnaire.pdf

Chapter 10
Planning recovery milestones

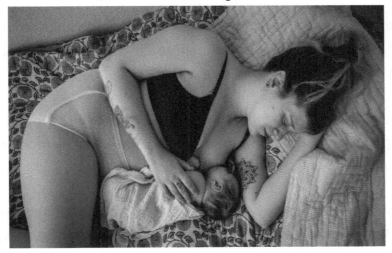

Why you should read this chapter:

- To help you anticipate milestones in your recovery and detect any deviations from normal.
- To help you plan your recovery period wisely and avoid complications.
- To understand the need to permit yourself to take time to return to pre-pregnancy activity.
- Recommendations for resuming sexual relationships and contraceptive choices.

Transition to motherhood

This central rite of passage into motherhood requires a helping hand (excuse the pun) to support women in their body's recovery and re-acclimatisation, knowing it would go a long way to enhancing a healthy, happy postpartum surgical recovery. The transition from hospital to community opens a whole new postoperative experience for the surgically delivered mother; her journey and recovery from birth are very different from vaginal birth. In previous chapters, we have explored hurdles of recovery, including pain management, wound healing, and supporting breast or bottle-feeding. The spiritual transition to motherhood and parenting is also an important consideration at this life-changing time and the huge responsibility that comes with being responsible for nurturing a new little life.

In the busyness of the early hours and days following birth, you can miss the early warning signs and symptoms of ill health, maternal mental health demise, feeding and breastfeeding difficulties, and wound care issues.

We advise you to take time to reflect, be mindful of what you have just experienced, including the pregnancy journey you have been on. We would never get into a car and drive it without lessons and be safe without a test.

Transition to parenting is going to be just like that. A process of ups and downs including likes and dislikes, fatigue, joy, and lows. Before you know it, days have turned into weeks, and your transition, strength, capabilities, and routines will develop.

Our top tip in this phase of transition into becoming a mother and parent is to relax, rest, and sleep when a baby sleeps to restore your energy levels.

Check out—Caesarcare's gift suggestions for mums offer some great ideas: <https://www.caesarcare.com/blog/8-practical-gift-ideas-for-c-section-mums>.

Healing in body, mind, and spirit
We are three-dimensional beings, and we need to pay attention to all three, finding whatever ways to best strengthen and enliven your mind, body, and spirit, for example, meditation, exercise, nature walks, music, yoga, prayer, journaling, laughter, and singing.

Figure 10.1 Postpartum healing

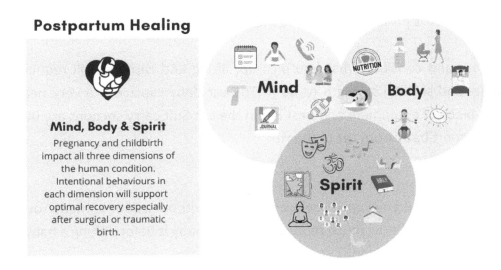

L Rastas 2020

Postpartum emotions

Emotions can fluctuate if you are concerned about changes in your mental state; it is wise to talk it out with a healthcare professional. Chapter 9, 'Maternal mental health—how am I supposed to feel?', is worth a revisit if you find your emotional state in tatters. We ask you to remember that tiredness and fatigue will contribute to your emotional recovery.

You will benefit from extra help from family or friends within your home in the early recovery days. Their help with simple chores like washing, cooking a healthy meal, and cleaning will help you refocus your emotional energy. Regular power naps, again, are powerful energy restorers, and we recommend you sleep when the baby sleeps to restore your dynamic balances.

How much is too heavy?

Remember not to lift anything heavier than your baby in the first six weeks of recovery.

As explored in Chapter 2, wound recovery is more profound than the skin scar. Five abdominal layers will take up to six weeks to knit back together. This milestone in your recovery journey is probably one of the most important.

Take it easy and consider what you pick up: lifting and carrying will require some abdominal and skeletal strength to do it. The car baby capsule is a very heavy and awkward piece of equipment and best left in the car. Soft carry cocoons are better for you to transport baby from car to pram.

Baby carriers

Most baby carriers already weigh between 5–10 kg without a baby in them. You should be more conscious of how much more weight your baby is before lifting a baby carrier during the postpartum period.

You are advised to get help with caring roles like bathing your baby.

Carrying any heavy load after abdominal surgery is not conserving your energy. It will put stress on abdominal tissue trying to heal and reconnect.

You might feel tired after surgery and will need to make the most of your energy. Lifting and strenuous activity like vacuuming or carrying wet laundry and grocery shopping is not advised. Your abdominal muscles also help protect your back, and if you strain these muscles, you may compromise your recovery.

We are not saying you cannot potter about and do some gentle activities like meal preparation, light dusting, and light laundry activities; we just ask you to be safe and allow yourself the time to recover.

Some lift handling tips:

- Assess the object before lifting, such as its size and weight.
- Bend at the knees to pick up the object.

- Avoid twisting when bending, lifting, or putting an object down.
- Carry the item in both hands.
- Hold the object close to you. You should avoid pushing and pulling activities, such as vacuuming, scrubbing the bath, hanging up heavy washing, and grocery shopping, carrying heavy bags.

Pacing, prioritising, and planning
Try the following:

- **Pacing:** spread tasks throughout the day and try not to cram everything into the morning.
- **Prioritising:** does it need to be done today?
- **Planning:** choose the best time of day for you to do your activities.

Getting back behind the wheel
You should ideally not drive a car until you have fully recovered and your wound has healed. Healing may take up to six weeks. Your obstetrician can provide advice about when it is safe to drive again.

The Drivers' Medical Unit at the Driving and Vehicle Licensing Agency (DVLA) suggests listening to your surgeon's advice. You should only drive again when you are free of pain and able to perform an emergency stop comfortably. You should check with your insurance company to make sure you are covered to start driving again.

Consider:

- Will my insurance cover me?
- Am I able to safely pick up the car seat and fix it without straining my abdomen, back, and wound?
- How alert am I?
- Can someone else help me?

Sexual intercourse

Whilst sex is probably the last thing on your mind postpartum, it will raise its head in the coming weeks as a topic to be explored and discussed.

It is naturally much safer to avoid penetrative sex until you feel comfortable, pain-free, all surgical sites are healing, and there is no vaginal bleeding. Infection and pain management will lead to this milestone in your recovery.

Sex, after either vaginal or surgical delivery, has become a postoperative topic women shrug off. Yet it is policy to discuss sex and contraception with women before discharge. This seems entirely reasonable to women as their body and emotional chemistry will be in overdrive. In our experience, the topic has always raised eyebrows! When speaking with women at six weeks postnatal reviews, it is the norm to hear them reflect that sexual activities have not resumed. This is often said with a glimmer of anticipated dread. This recovery period and choice will be a very individual decision and an experience that should not be forced or coerced. Many women have voiced throughout our clinical and community affairs that it took weeks to many months before they felt ready. Birth mode and birth traumas will undoubtedly take a toll on decisions around sexual activity.

Strenuous activity, including sex, can increase the risk of opening the incision.

Fear of causing damage can be a psychological barrier to intercourse, and recognition of this and finding ways to mitigate it will be important. Some women find hypnosis or mindfulness meditation and visualisation helpful in this area.

If the incision site is sore, try positions that do not put any pressure on the abdomen.

Painful sex, known as dyspareunia, can occur after any birth. It is essential to discuss with your doctor or physiotherapist if you are experiencing sexual health difficulties.

Creativity and partner understanding to find comfortable positions and other sensory relaxation and mindfulness techniques may also help restore you to full sexual health.[11]

Physical posture and stretches

Maintaining a good posture will help your wound heal and restore strength in your body. Repeat the following positions slowly. It is normal to feel a slight pulling sensation. Try to do them three times a day, gradually building up to five repetitions of each.

- Stretch 1: While standing, gently push your hips forward and lean backward.
- Stretch 2: While standing cross arms over chest, ease your torso left and right.
- Rotations: Cross your arms over your chest and clasp the opposite shoulder. Gently twist/rotate slowly to each side.

You can stop these stretches when you feel you are back to the level you were before the C-section.

When is a good time to start pelvic floor exercises?

Pelvic floor exercises are essential to do during pregnancy and as soon as you can post-delivery. You may not notice you are doing actual benefits at first, but attempt to do these simple exercises daily.

Your pelvic floor is a broad sling of muscles, ligaments, and sheet-like tissues that stretch from your pubic bone at the front of your body to the base of your spine at the back.

The pelvic floor is sometimes compared to a trampoline, as it can stretch down under pressure from weight and bounce up again.

However, if your pelvic floor muscles are weighed down for a long time, as they are during pregnancy, they can become weak, so they don't bounce back as far.

Weak pelvic floor muscles may make it harder for you to control your bladder, especially in your second and third trimesters. That's because a soft pelvic floor makes it harder for you to squeeze the muscles and sphincters at the bottom of your bladder to prevent urine from escaping.

The whole area between your anus and vagina (perineum) after birth is essential; weak muscles can lead to urinary and sexual problems.

Building strength in your pelvic floor muscles can help to:

- Support the extra weight of pregnancy.
- Protect you from leaking wee while you're pregnant and after your baby is born.
- Help your pelvis recover from birth is especially symphysis pubis dysfunction **(SPD).**
- Make for a more satisfying sex life by increasing sensation.
- Prevent a prolapse.

How to do pelvic floor exercises?
For over twenty years, this simple, effective set of instructions we have used in care plans with women has supported their awareness and use of pelvic floor exercises.

First, make sure you can feel your pelvic floor muscles. You can do this by squeezing and lifting the muscles around your urethra, vagina, and anus. Imagine bringing your tail bone towards your pubic bone and all the muscles helping to draw forward.

Imagine you're trying to stop urinating midstream, at the same time as gripping a tampon with your vagina and preventing yourself from passing wind.

The muscles you can feel contracting on the inside of your pelvis are the muscles you're aiming to strengthen. You should squeeze hard enough to feel a little trembling in your vagina. If you pull hard enough, you may also engage your lower tummy muscles tightening just above your groin. It's a subtle sensation, but it will become more apparent as you get used to doing the exercises.

Notice the difference between when your muscles are tight and when they are relaxed. At first, it's enough to hold the squeeze for a few seconds, then release as you get used to the feel of your muscles contracting and relaxing.

It's more important to exercise the right muscles for a little time than to apply the wrong forces for longer. For example, your tummy shouldn't contract above your belly button, and you shouldn't squeeze your inner thighs and buttocks.

When you first try pelvic floor exercises, if you can't feel anything when you try them while sitting, work them while lying down. Lie on your side if you're later on in pregnancy, as this is safer for your baby and more comfortable for you.

Lying down to do your exercises may help you get a feel for where your muscles are. Once you know how to do the exercises in this position, doing them while standing will become easier. Making a cup of tea or when doing a nappy change are ideal times to practice pelvic floor muscles.

Pelvic muscle exercises
- Squeeze and hold for ten seconds, then relax for a few seconds. Repeat ten times. This long, ten-second squeeze helps to support your growing baby and your bladder and bowel.
- Follow your set of ten long squeezes with ten short squeezes. The short squeezes will help you control your bladder when you cough, exercise, or sneeze.
- Do this set of ten long and ten short squeezes three times a day. Keep in mind 'ten, ten, three' to remind you of your daily target.

Remember that 'ten, ten, three' is your target. If you're not used to exercising your pelvic floor, five squeezes five times a day is sufficient to start. Build up to ten as soon as you're able.

When you first try pelvic floor exercises, you may find that you hold your breath as you squeeze. You'll need to learn to breathe as you do the exercises. When you cough or sneeze, you breathe out forcefully. If you can only tighten your muscles when you hold your breath, they will relax when you cough or sneeze, and you may leak wee.

After a few months, you should start to notice your pelvic floor exercises making a difference. Try not to get disheartened if you can't feel much, though. Your baby is getting bigger all the time, which means your pelvic floor will have to work harder to support your womb. Keep going, as your efforts will pay off.

Don't worry if you start to exercise them later in pregnancy than you'd have liked. Start as soon as you can. Continue doing the exercises after birth. It's just as essential to help your pelvic area recover. Pelvic floor exercises need to be a habit for life! If you have vaginal trauma, we advise allowing a few days of healing time to allow any swelling or suturing to ease. A swollen perineum and anal haemorrhoids can all prevent you from starting a new recovery exercise.

<https://www.ouh.nhs.uk/patient-guide/leaflets/files/4895Pchildbirth.pdf>
<https://www.thewomens.org.au/images/uploads/fact-sheets/Pelvic-floor-exercises-210319.pdf>

When can I start workouts after surgery, and how can I gain strength?
As you gain confidence, strength, and wellbeing, you can reduce the likelihood of complications if you wait until after six weeks. Five layers need to heal, and they take up to six weeks to heal internally.

Gentle exercise as described above is recommended until then.

Useful tips to strengthen your legs and arms remain essential; take more care with abdominal and vaginal muscles.

What activity can I safely do?
Posture/stretching and pelvic floor exercises only are recommended for six weeks.

Jogging can be painful
Soreness in the incision site is a sign your body is not ready. Back off. Do not be a frustrated jogger.

Wounds healing and pain subsiding?
Pain should subside with healing; remember, five layers are healing, so take our advice: do it gradually, and do not cause internal damage too soon.

First, second, third, and fourth-degree vaginal tears
If you laboured and were unfortunate also to get vaginal tearing or have an episiotomy, then having a caesarean on top of this means there is a lot to heal. A summary of these tears follows:

- First-degree tear: tear involving the perineal or vaginal skin only.
- Second-degree tear: perineal skin and muscles are torn, but intact anal sphincter.
- Third-degree perineal tear: perineal skin, muscles, and anal sphincter is involved.
  - Less than 50% of the external anal sphincter thickness is damaged.
  - More than 50% of the external anal sphincter thickness is damaged, but the internal anal sphincter intact.
  - Both external and internal anal sphincters are damaged, but anal mucosa intact.
- Fourth-degree perineal tear: perineal skin, muscles, anal sphincter, and anal mucosa is damaged.
- Button-hole tear: anal sphincter is intact, but anal mucosa is damaged.

Anatomically, an episiotomy involves the same structures as a second-degree perineal tear. Tears in labour are standard, and an attempt to vaginally deliver could have resulted in either of these tears or an episiotomy (cut).

These tears occur in the perineum and can extend to the anus in a third-degree tear.

The tears and cuts often occur due to fast birth, shoulder dystocia, forceps, and ventouse; big babies can tear the vaginal wall in a vaginal attempt to deliver.

These tears will take up to eight weeks to recover, and pelvic floor exercise is essential to recovery. Sexual intercourse after a second, third, or fourth-degree tear can cause pain and discomfort. Couples should wait until healing is complete. And in the early days of resuming sexual intercourse, the use of a lubricant is recommended.

Contraceptive choices

There are about thirteen types and choices for women and two options for men. In most countries, post-birth contraception is free for up to a year after delivery. Contraception choices after a caesarean birth are extra important. Full internal healing is advised after surgery, so taking a moment to explore and find out your options is essential to your recovery and future reproductive choices ahead of you.[74]

Sterilisation methods

Sterilisation involves a surgical procedure to prevent pregnancy permanently. These are vasectomy for males and tubal ligation or occlusion for females. Female sterilisation includes a permanent procedure to prevent pregnancy. This is also called tubal ligation or 'getting your tubes tied'. It is a permanent form of birth control. The fallopian tubes are cut, sealed, clipped, or tied. After consultation and consent, at C-section, sterilisation procedures are performed.[75]

How do I choose a method?

There are many contraception methods and natural family planning methods to choose from, and it's worth taking the time to find out more about each one so that you can select the method that suits you; these include the following methods.

Natural methods for avoiding conception

There are nine natural methods to try to avoid pregnancy: calendar rhythm method, basal body temperature method, mucus inspection method, symptothermal method, ovulation prediction testing kits, withdrawal method, lactational infertility (breastfeeding) method, douching and urination, and abstinence.

- Lactational amenorrhoea method (LAM): Breastfeeding can give rise to lactational amenorrhoea and can be effective in preventing pregnancy, providing a woman meets the following criteria:
  - gave birth less than six months ago
  - breastfeeding exclusively including a night feed (no formula or solid food)
  - Hasn't had a period since giving birth.

The risk of pregnancy during lactational infertility is 1 in 50: <https://www.breastfeeding.asn.au/bfinfo/lactational-amenorrhea-method-lam-postpartum-contraception>.

Intrauterine devices

Long-acting reversible contraceptives. These provide birth control with a three- to ten-year lifespan. Examples are intrauterine devices and hormonal implants, and injections.

Oral contraceptives

Short-acting hormonal methods include birth control that you take every day or month like the pill, mini pills, patch, and vaginal ring. There's also a shot that your doctor can administer every three months.

Barrier methods

Used each time you have sex, barrier methods are condoms, diaphragms, sponges, and cervical caps.

- Most contraception methods won't protect you against catching or passing on sexually transmitted infections (STI). Condoms are the only method that can protect against both STI and pregnancy.

Your choice and your partners will help support an active, healthy sex life.

Six weeks postnatal

Find out about your postnatal check. Not all locality services do them.[76] It is, however, good practice to get medically checked out after C-section birth. At this time, contraceptive choices can be discussed, including reviewing your maternal mental health, physical and social, and emotional aspects of care.

Cervical smears

Cervical screening (a smear test) is available to women aged twenty-five to sixty-four years.

The cervix or opening to your womb is examined for cancer and cell changes.

Taking part in the National Cervical Screening service can reduce the incidence of and mortality from cervical cancer by a systematic, quality assured population-based screening.[77] Cervical screening can be a lifesaver; we advise you do not miss your invitations to be screened.

Weight loss after pregnancy and birth

Losing weight after having a baby for many women is a struggle.

How much to lose and when to lose it is essential, especially if you are breastfeeding.

Most women will lose at least five kilograms during childbirth, including the placenta, weight of the baby, and amniotic fluid.

During the first six weeks after surgery, your body needs rest and plenty of nutrition for healing your internal and external wounds.

If you are breastfeeding, you will need at least 500 calories/2092 kJ a day to produce breast milk. The tip is to stay healthy, drink water sensibly, and eat a proper, well-balanced diet. Avoid extra sugars from takeaway, soft drink, and junk food.

Reclaiming your body will take a while; check out this site for top tips: <https://www.healthline.com/nutrition/weight-loss-after-pregnancy>.

Dealing with stretch marks

One thing about stretch marks: they are not preventable!

Considering the cause of stretch marks is tearing deep beneath the skin, it shouldn't come as too much of a surprise that there's no tried-and-true cure. It's impossible to 100 percent get rid of your stretch marks, but don't be too discouraged—there are steps you can take to reduce their appearance, namely by rebuilding the collagen in your skin with some excellent counter products and a committed skincare routine. But do not use any products on unhealed skin.

Your suture scar line will take up to eight weeks to recover.

Date night and time out from parenting

Whether you plan to celebrate the birth of your baby, your anniversary, or escape the baby for the night, date night needs to be on your couple-reconnecting calendar.

Be creative and realistic; there will be much planning involved, and choose when you are likely not to fall asleep at the restaurant table.

Reconnect and remind yourselves that baby came to live with you, not the other way round.

Going out with a baby

Planning a day out with a baby is a mammoth task at first. There seems to be so much equipment to take with you: nappies, food, change of clothing, steriliser, baby nest, pram, etc. Here are some tips:

- Make a list; keep it simple.
- Decide how long you need to be out.
- Think about the activity.
- Don't forget the forgettable.

The first days out are exciting milestones. Be safe and enjoy it but return if you feel tired or stressed. Build up your confidence, and eventually, you will be hanging out with the other mammas soon.

Car seats and safety

How to choose the right car seat for your baby will depend upon your car, its fixings, its size, and the baby's weight.

Remember it is going to get heavier, so choose wisely. In the early days, do not be the one to insist on carrying the baby in a carrier. We have discussed they can often weigh 5–10 kg without a baby!

It is probably the most safety-conscious product you will ever buy your child, and there will be more than one to choose from.

Car seat safety laws to adhere to their safety is paramount at all times, even in a pram. Take a browse through ROSPA UK safety tips to choose wisely and safely.[78] ROSPA do not advise buying a second-hand car seat—you may be purchasing a lethal carrier.

Australian car seat safety guidelines can be found at <https://www.childcarseats.com.au/legal-requirements> <https://www.childcarseats.org.uk/>.

Summary

Chapter 10 has explored the recovery milestones that women want to achieve by six weeks postnatal in our experience.

It's natural to long for your flat stomach back without any scars or stretch marks after delivering your baby. The transition to motherhood has taken its toll; healing physically and emotionally will take some hurdle-jumping to recover fully. It is essential to approach your postpartum fitness routine with caution, especially if you've had a C-section birth. A C-section birth is major abdominal surgery, and your body needs as much time as possible to recover.

Reflecting on the topics, we have discussed, like lifting, resting, power naps, pelvic floor exercises, are all preparation for restoring you, restoring your health to make choices about sexual health and contraception, and all-important use of trusted sitters for date night. Getting you to the six-week postpartum milestone of continued recovery depends on you; your support network is there to help you recover and stay well. Important screening like cervical smears will support long term health needs and reproductive health.

Even simple choices you make on child safety seats, how you lift them, when you drive, and return to physical activities are all as important as feeding your baby.

Putting yourself first means you can recover fitness levels in a timely manner.

You know your body and set your own recovery milestones by using the daily planner as an indicator for wellbeing.

- Each day of each week will help track your recovery.
- Using a mantra we both used with mothers is a great reminder:
  'It took you nine months to grow a baby; see how you recover within nine months'.

References

74. FPA Contraceptive Choices https://www.fpa.org.uk/sites/default/files/your-guide-to-contraception.pdf

75. NHS Female sterilisation retrieved from https://www.nhs.uk/conditions/contraception/female-sterilisation/

76. https://www.nhs.uk/conditions/pregnancy-and-baby/postnatal-check/

77. https://cks.nice.org.uk/cervical-screening

78. https://www.rospa.com/lets-talk-about/2017/February/New-child-car-seat-laws

Chapter 11
Challenges related to C-section birth and pregnancy

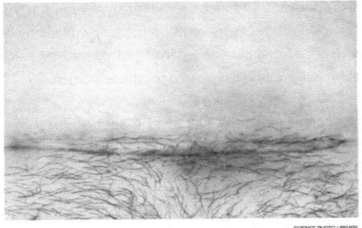

Why you should read this chapter:

- To appreciate the importance of good preparation and reflection.
- To understand the potential challenges of caesarean birth and recovery.
- To be aware of considerations for any subsequent pregnancies—including vaginal birth after caesarean (VBAC).
- To appreciate the impact of co-existing medical conditions on pregnancy.

Sophie's story

Whilst my first was a forty-two-hour labour and emergency section, this time we only just made it to the hospital. I had never contemplated VBAC, but I did it with just gas and air, and I'm so glad I did because the recovery afterwards was much easier, especially with a three-year-old at home!

Having a C-section can have a significant impact on a mother's mental and physical health in the weeks afterward. To speed up your recovery, you can try various lifestyle and wellness methods. With recovery comes a challenge; planning how to deal with any difficulties have been listed here, taken from postoperative C-section women and midwives and health visitors who have cared for these women.

What is placenta accreta and the risk after C-section?

Placenta accreta is an obstetric condition where the placenta grows more firmly into the uterine wall. There are varying degrees and could carry an obstetric haemorrhage risk. Accreta increases with the number of C-sections you have. It is more complicated with a pregnancy with placenta praevia (placental covering the womb opening).[79]

Infertility after C-section

After a C-section, scar tissue, including adhesions, is normal. However, some internal scar tissue can build up over the reproductive organs and, in some cases, cause infertility problems.[80]

Failed anaesthetic, haemorrhage

Learn about the risks, recovery time, and anaesthetic choices for this procedure.

If you had an emergency C-section, it was because your life or your baby's life was in danger and vaginal birth was no longer an option. Seconds count when making obstetric choices; this includes the option of anaesthetic. Epidural, a spinal block, or a general anaesthetic all carry risks; if the epidural or spinal block fails, then a general anaesthetic will be given.

C-section is major abdominal surgery that involves the management of several personnel. Haemorrhaging and reactions to anaesthetic go hand in hand with that risk. This is why, in emergency C-section situations, patient consent forms are rapidly signed and leave little time to discuss all the pros and cons of surgery. Emergency situations call for safety and speed to secure the wellbeing of mother and baby.

How many C-sections can I have?

A caesarean birth is classified as major surgery that carries several risks, so it's usually only done if it's the safest option for you and your baby.

Each one will become more complicated, for sure, as the risk of so much scar tissue on the abdomen and uterus will add the risk of complications.

There are safety recommendations, but generally, it's desirable to be in good health. When you conceive a subsequent pregnancy, you will be treated as a high-risk pregnancy. This is primarily as some options previously open to you may be reduced once you have a history of caesarean birth.

The historical recommendation is generally no more than three caesarean births, however, this should be assessed on an individual basis due to the risks associated. There are many social media support groups for C-section mums and many women have had many more than three C-sections, some as many as ten or more. Healing from C-section, whatever type of scar, is paramount, as is the timing of the next pregnancy. Periods of a year or more allow the five layers to heal and your anatomy and physical wellbeing to return to a safer level.

Effect of classic or inverted T-scar on subsequent pregnancies

Each scar will carry a small degree of risk of rupture. The American College of Obstetricians and Gynaecologists (ACOG) state that individual circumstances should be considered in all cases. Valuable research articles and case studies can be found at 'Special scars' to help you better make decisions for subsequent pregnancies.[81]

What are the risks of vaginal birth after caesarean (VBAC)?

Whilst uterine rupture—though very rare—is the major risk, there are very few reasons why you would not plan to have a VBAC. To help with your decision, see the discussion in the ACOG Practice Bulletin for the 2017 ACOG practice guidelines. VBAC can be a safe and empowering and healing experience for many women.[82]

It is important that you get evidence-based advice when deciding on your trial of labour after caesarean (TOLAC) as women can be discouraged by unfounded advice and opinions. Seek out midwifery practices that support TOLAC to discuss your wishes. Research by Australian midwife and VBAC researcher Hazel Keedle found that women who had continuity of care with a midwife felt more in control, had more confidence, were more likely to have an upright labour and birth, and had a relationship based on equity, trust, and support, compared to continuity of care with a doctor or standard antenatal care.[83]

You should make an informed choice based on your health, recovery, and general wellbeing before getting pregnant again. Five layers will take up to a year to heal and recover. What you see on the outside is just the skin layer of your body—remember there are four other layers internally.

Hazel's story

My first birth was a planned homebirth which went very far from the plan! I was hospitalised with pneumonia at 34 weeks for a week and then went into spontaneous labour after my waters rupturing at 37 weeks. My little boy was confirmed as breech presentation during labour, and I was transferred to a hospital with a no vaginal breech birth policy, and I had an emergency caesarean. About a week later, I was back in hospital with endometritis!

I didn't do great both physically and emotionally after those experiences. When my baby boy was around six months old, I noticed breastfeeding was becoming sore, and I did a pregnancy test. I was shocked to find out I was pregnant, and an ultrasound showed I was about two months pregnant. This sent me into a hive of reading about VBAC and I learnt that the uterine risk rupture risk did increase for a shorter interpregnancy period, but only to 2%, which meant I had a 98% chance of no uterine rupture. As a midwife, I did avoid a lot of antenatal care by getting my colleagues to check my blood pressure and baby's heart rate. I did plan a VBAC at home, but when I went into labour at 38 weeks, my support team couldn't be there, so I transferred to a large hospital about forty-five mins from home.

During labour, I had a lot of negativities from a couple of the midwives and the doctor that kept coming in to try to persuade me to go for a repeat caesarean. I was told I was too quiet and then too loud and that I should stay on the bed! I think I was left alone a lot, which was better for me, but I did get my hubby to call a colleague friend who was relieved off her work to come and support me. She talked me through my transitional doubts, and I dug deep for even more strength as I felt my baby descend and start the involuntary pushing stage! She got me a birthing stool as I was trying to squat, and my hubby sat behind me holding onto me. That was very helpful as the doctor came in saying I must get on the bed and a couple of midwives tried to pick me up. My husband is a big and strong man, and they had no hope! At the time, they threatened to take me to theatre, I roared my baby out of my vagina and onto my chest! I did it! I pushed her out of my vagina!

Having a VBAC was a monumental moment for me; it was healing and empowering but left me with many questions about other women's experiences. That led me to become a VBAC researcher and complete a PhD in women's experiences of planning a VBAC in Australia!

How long will I bleed for after birth?

Postpartum bleeding after birth can generally last ten to twenty-one days. It will change in colour from bright red to dark red. After too much exercise, you may see more bleeding. It should not run or drip from you.

You should wear clean pads often and observe your loss, reporting any concerns of excess to your medical support team.

It is a good idea to pour warm water over yourself at each toilet session; this will douche your perineal area and avoid any unwanted smell. Wear external pads, not internal tampons.

Passing clots/retained placental deposits

Postpartum bleeding can be a worry; each woman will bleed differently. Do not worry if you pass small clots, as long as they are smaller than a golf ball.

Larger clots are of some concern as you may be pooling blood. Speak to your health care professional and keep and show any clot you pass.

Change your pad regularly, stay clean, and if there are any smaller undelivered placental deposits, then other symptoms are likely. These can include uterine cramps, offensive smell, pain, generally feeling unwell, and clots. As the body tries to expel this, your symptoms may change, you can experience pain and feel unwell.

In some cases, retained placental deposits can be the cause and need removal in the hospital. Some women report cramps to be like labour pains—this is a common description as the uterus will contract to try to expel any debris, like placenta deposits or blood clots. Get advice from your medical team if you suspect this. Retained products of conception are one of the leading causes of postpartum haemorrhage and infection.

Hysterectomy at C-section

Postpartum hysterectomy (removal of the uterus) is associated with complications during the procedure. Certain conditions like life-threatening haemorrhaging will lead to this.

Removal of the uterus will mean you can no longer get pregnant.[84]

Gestational diabetes/Diabetes Mellitus

This is a condition where high blood sugar (glucose) develops during pregnancy. You will undergo screening for this if it is suspected. It usually disappears after birth.

It can increase the likelihood of the pregnancy being complicated, and the baby growing more substantial in size, resulting in the need for a C-section.

Some women may need to eat a sugar-free diet, check their blood sugars, or even take insulin injections.

You cannot prevent it, but you can eat sensibly. It is an endocrine complication. You can develop it again in future pregnancies, and this needs regular close monitoring.[85]

Diabetes Mellitus may be a pre-existing condition that will have the same potential complications.

Pre-eclampsia

Pre-eclampsia is a disorder of pregnancy that presents as a complication, requiring close medical monitoring.

It can lead to high blood pressure, protein in the urine, abdominal pain, spots before your eye, headaches, swollen limbs, fingers, feet, reduced baby movements, fitting, and in severe cases, stillbirth, or maternal and foetal death.[86]

Urine samples at antenatal visits help detect this condition and blood pressure reviews. Tell your medical team if you present with any symptoms from about twenty weeks into your pregnancy.

It is a severe condition, and you need to see your medical team if you present with any symptoms.

In severe cases, delivering the baby can be the only safe cure for mothers, depending on the gestation of the baby this can happen too early to save a baby.

Cholestasis

Intrahepatic cholestasis of pregnancy (ICP) is a severe liver disorder that can develop in pregnancy. Bile acids become impaired from leaving the body.

Women complain of drowsiness, whole body itching and scratching, fatigue, and can often suffer jaundice (skin/whites of eyes turn yellow).[87]

Seek medical attention if you have any symptoms.

Cholestasis in severe cases can lead to early delivery of a baby and high morbidity, and the pregnancy and baby's movements must be monitored very closely.

Symphysis pubis dysfunction (SPD)

Pelvic-related pain in pregnancy. It is reported to be very painful and can be debilitating enough to use crutches to mobilise.

It happens when the pelvic ligaments, the ligaments that usually keep your pelvic bone aligned during pregnancy, become too relaxed and stretchy too soon, resulting in pain and difficulty mobilising.[88]

Pain relief and physiotherapy is recommended. In severe cases, it can impede a vaginal delivery.

Reduced foetal movements

Report any reduced baby movements to your medical team. Your baby should kick and move from around sixteen weeks gestation. If you notice a reduction in your baby's movements, get checked out by your medical team.

Remember, counting the kicks can be a lifesaver.[89]

Your baby's health can be monitored by its movements. Women must be encouraged to become 'in tune' with baby movements so they can detect any early warning signs.

Maternal obesity

Maternal obesity increases the risk of several pregnancy complications, including pre-eclampsia, gestational diabetes, C-section, wound infection, and more. Maternal size can be associated with many birth complications. Eat healthy, exercise, and take advice if you feel you have an increased BMI. Raising the issue of weight in pregnancy is essential; it is a measure of wellbeing.

In our experience, both vaginal births and C-sections can be complicated by maternal obesity.

Smoking in pregnancy/smoking and cot death

Every cigarette or vaping carries chemicals to your baby passing through the placental membrane and causing harm to you and your unborn baby. Tobacco can restrict the flow of oxygen through the placenta to your baby.

Key points to think about:

- You decided to smoke, not your baby.
- Your baby will be affected by smoking.

- Your baby could be small for gestation.
- Second-hand smoking is unsafe. Do not inhale secondary smoke.
- Low birth-weight babies are more likely to have complications.
- Smoking increases the risk of miscarriage.
- Smoking can increase the risk of stillbirth.
- Smoking around a baby can increase the chances of cot death.
- Smoking decreases healthy tissue repair.

Know the risks. Seek smoking cessation support and give your baby a fighting chance.[90]

Alcohol and pregnancy

Drinking alcohol during pregnancy puts your unborn baby at risk as well as you. There is no safe level of alcohol consumption during pregnancy. Health advice also recommends alcohol should not be consumed when trying to conceive or breastfeed. There are many serious side effects from drinking alcohol.

Some of the most serious risks of exposing your unborn baby to alcohol are:

- slowed baby growth
- low birth weight
- premature birth
- miscarriage (losing a baby before 24 weeks of pregnancy)
- stillbirth (a baby being born dead after 24 weeks of pregnancy)
- a range of physical, mental, behavioural, and learning disabilities that are collectively called fetal alcohol spectrum disorder (FASD).

Read more at <https://www.betterhealth.vic.gov.au/health/healthyliving/Alcohol-and-pregnancy#bhc-content> and <https://www.nhs.uk/pregnancy/keeping-well/drinking-alcohol-while-pregnant/>.

Obstructed birth

Obstructed vaginal birth is when the baby cannot progress to be born vaginally.[91]

Postpartum Haemorrhage/Primary

Postpartum haemorrhage (PPH) is more bleeding than average after the birth of your baby. About one in 100 women will have a postpartum haemorrhage after C-section.

A PPH is when you lose more than 500 mL of blood within the first twenty-four hours.

How could a PPH affect me?

If you lose a lot of blood, it can worsen the normal tiredness that all women feel after having a baby. If heavy bleeding does occur, it is essential to treat it quickly. Significant bleeding can be life-threatening.

Who is at risk? Risk factors for primary PPH before the birth

- having had a PPH in a previous pregnancy
- BMI>35
- having had four or more babies
- carrying twins or triplets
- ethnicity
- having a low-lying placenta (placenta praevia)
- the placenta coming away early (placental abruption)
- pre-eclampsia, and high blood pressure
- anaemia in labour
- birth by caesarean section
- induction of labour
- retained placenta
- episiotomy (a vaginal cut to help birth)
- forceps or ventouse birth
- labouring for more than twelve hours
- having a big baby (more than 4kgs/9lbs)
- having your first baby if you are more than forty years old.

The risk factors and the incidence of PPH are associated but not always a cause.

Secondary PPH occurs (after the birth)

- When you have abnormal or heavy vaginal bleeding between twenty-four hours and twelve weeks after the birth. It affects fewer than 2 in 100 women.
- A secondary PPH is often associated with infection and usually occurs after you have left the hospital. You should contact your midwife or GP if your bleeding is getting more substantial or if your lochia has an offensive smell. You are likely to be given a course of antibiotics. Any heavy bleeding or concerns, you should seek medical advice.
- Retained placental tissue needs to be removed and will require hospitalisation. You may need antibiotics through a drip and less commonly an operation to clear your uterus of any infection, blood clots, or small pieces of placenta that remain retained after your baby was born need to be expelled. Your baby can usually stay with you if you wish, and you can continue to breastfeed even if you are taking antibiotics.[92]

Kangaroo babies/babywearing
Babywearing simply means carrying your baby in a sling or baby carrier.

Birth takes its toll on your body, as does pregnancy, for that matter. Still, a caesarean birth is different as you have all of the usual factors involved after birth, but also the added complication of major abdominal surgery recovery.

Lots of people ask us when they can first use a sling after a C-section. The answer is when you feel ready.

In all aspects of carrying especially while pregnant or recently after birth, we strongly advise you to listen to your body, do what is comfortable, and build up to more extended periods, if you wish to, just as crucial with a C-section.

Summary

Your plans and challenges can be reduced if you make wise choices when choosing your maternal healthcare.

Be sure you get the answers to three key questions:

1. What are my options?
2. What are the pros and cons of each option for me?
3. How do I get support to help me make a decision that is right for me? [93]

We began this chapter by stating: 'With recovery comes a challenge.' Planning how to deal with any challenges is now your decision, your choice, and your recovery. Overcoming any challenge is the first step to recovery. Helping you understand how you plan and prepare your recovery and future reproductive health is part of our legacy to you so that you can make informed choices. This chapter should help in some way support you with answers to the *why*, *what*, *when*, and *how* you resulted in having a C-section birth. Making sure you become you again should help you to know you are not alone, but you do have the information to own your recovery journey.

References

79. RANZCOG (2021) Placenta Accreta retrieved from https://ranzcog.edu.au/RANZCOG_SITE/media/RANZCOG-

80. NHS (2021)Planning another pregnancy. https://www.nhs.uk/conditions/pregnancy-and-baby/planning-another-pregnancy/

81. Specialscars.(2020) retrieved from http://specialscars.org

82. American College of Obstetricians and Gynaecologists ACOG (2020) VBAC guidelines -retrieved from https://www.aafp.org/afp/2004/1001/p1397.html

83. Keedle, H., Peters, L., Schmied, V. et al. (2020). Women's experiences of planning a vaginal birth after caesarean in different models of maternity care in Australia. BMC Pregnancy Childbirth 20, 381 https://doi.org/10.1186/s12884-020-03075-8

84. NHS Conditions. Retrieved from https://www.nhs.uk/conditions/hysterectomy/

85. From https://www.gestationaldiabetes.co.uk/

86. From https://www.nhs.uk/conditions/pre-eclampsia/

87. From https://www.nhs.uk/conditions/pregnancy-and-baby/itching-obstetric-cholestasis-pregnant/

88. From https://www.nhs.uk/conditions/pregnancy-and-baby/pelvic-pain-pregnant-spd/

89. Count the kicks App: https://www.countthekicks.org/app-download/

90. From https://www.who.int/tobacco/media/en/mitchell.pdf?ua=1; https://www.nhs.uk/conditions/pregnancy-and-baby/reducing-risk-cot-death/

91. From https://www.who.int/healthinfo/statistics/bod_obstructedlabour.pdf

92. From https://www.rcog.org.uk/globalassets/documents/patients/patient-information-leaflets/pregnancy/pi-heavy-bleeding-after-birth-postpartum-haemorrhage.pdf

93. Shepherd et al. (2011) Three questions that patients can ask to improve the quality of information physicians give about treatment options: A cross-over trial Patient Educ Couns. 2011 Sep;84(3):379-85. doi: 10.1016/j.pec.2011.07.022. Epub 2011 Aug 9. PMID: 21831558.

Chapter 12
Closing words—where to next?

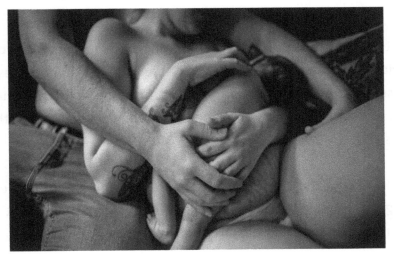

Comprehensive help should be given to mothers to aid their recovery; it is not acceptable to resign them to the narrative 'take it easy' after a C-section and simply expect them to get on with it.

There are sound reasons behind this narrative that require further explanation; women need to relate to and understand what is required to recover physically, mentally, and spiritually for optimum recovery. Knowing why we do what we do, and when we do it, forms the basis and impetus for good self-management and recovery.

All maternity care roles need to support the art and skill of birthing when caring for women. Each woman is an individual with individual histories, needs, and desires. Mothers, partners, children, and whole families require commitment to support their individual and public health and wellbeing.

If the first 1,001 days of a child's life can be shaped by the parent-child relationship focused on bonding and attachment, then the transition to parenthood must include further investment in 'how that child was born' and 'how well its parent was supported to nurture that relationship and their own maternal recovery'.

From conception through the first three years of life, parental bond is crucial in shaping a child's foundation for life.[94]

Emphasising the importance of birth method and birth recovery is captured in the words of a mother who agreed to tell her compelling story in our latest Five Guide postpartum sepsis prevention video: 'Families must be valued in their opinions, professionals, whoever that mum might be in contact with, will look at their wounds, and think sepsis!'

Dr Ron Daniels, CEO of the UK Sepsis Trust, reports: 'women are prone to infection following surgery.' He says, 'it is vital we look after women and spot the signs of infection and make appropriate referrals to prevent sepsis.'[95]

We hope *Your Body, Your Recovery* fulfils our quest to equip you to understand the *why*, *when*, *how*, and *what* happened to you and your body.

In three distinctive sections, we aimed to cover all the trade-learnt personal and professional experiences we have been privileged to be part of over eighty-five years collectively.

We hope you felt at times that you had your own virtual midwife with you.

Part One included twelve chapters as listed below, dedicated and chosen specifically as these have been the most challenging topics women and their families experience. In addition, throughout the book, we have curated stories from parents and birth partners to highlight the variety of experiences in relation to caesarean birth.

- Chapter 1: What is a caesarean section birth?
- Chapter 2: Five Guide—a tool to support your understanding of C-sections
- Chapter 3: The birth debrief—why it is so helpful?
- Chapter 4: Controlling your pain
- Chapter 5: Leaving hospital and adjusting to home
- Chapter 6: Mastering the art and skill of feeding baby
- Chapter 7: Safe sleeping and managing a crying baby
- Chapter 8: What do I need to know about my scar?
- Chapter 9: Maternal mental health—how am I supposed to feel?
- Chapter 10: Planning recovery milestones
- Chapter 11: Challenges related to C-section birth and pregnancy
- Chapter 12: Closing words—where to next?

Each one is dedicated to helping you and your body recover. We hope this manual helps you understand the anatomy and physiology of your caesarean birth and why specific care is recommended.

Part Two contains blank journals aimed at supporting your spiritual journey and debriefing journalling—a place to record, draw on, and secure your most precious feelings, photos, drawings, and many more doodling or thoughts you want to record.

Finally, Part Three recommends the use of forty-two (six weeks) daily planners which have the potential to help you navigate your recovery journey, your pain, your medication and act as time logs to help you keep track of your milestones during your postpartum period. The scar tracker and videos along the way are included to support you on your journey to recovery.

The joys and challenges of childbirth and parenting are many, and we hope that this manual has helped you to surmount the problems and to experience an abundance of joy, despite the pain of recovery.

Share it, keep it, review and reflect upon your entries, recommend it, or even buy it for a sister, a friend, or another mother you know would benefit from having it.

We feel privileged to be able to contribute to your healing and recovery as you transition into the incredible journey that is motherhood.

Thank you for trusting us to share our experience, love, and passion for helping mothers who birth their babies by caesarean section.

We firmly believe being informed is best and trust the information contained within has equipped you and empowered you for your best possible recovery.

May you continue to pay attention to nourishing your mind, body, and spirit daily and to become the best version of you and the best mother you can be.

With much love and blessings,
Janine & Leonie.

References

94. From https://www.nspcc.org.uk/globalassets/documents/news/critical-days-manifesto.pdf

95. From https://www.youtube.com/watch?v=cphHeFQvVxY

Part Two
Journal Pages

Introduction to Maternal Journalling

Becoming a mother is a transformative experience and an ever-evolving journey, with no two days the same.

Journalling can be a good way to help you observe your progress as you begin your journey. There will be good days and bad days after caesarean birth, and these pages give you permission to celebrate or pour out your frustrations using whatever medium best suits you. Taking time to reflect and document your story can be a wonderful gift to yourself as you grow as a mother and heal from your major surgery. Journalling is good for you—physically, mentally, and emotionally.

Five powerful benefits of journalling

Reduces stress

Improves immune function

Keeps memory sharp

Boosts mood

Strengthens emotional functions

Some ways you may find helpful to express your story

A short story

A sketch

Painting

Gratitude points

Dreams

Creating a checklist

Listing achievements big and small

A place to communicate your needs

You will find optional prompts at the top of each page and encouraging quotes at the foot.

Prompt

The best part of my day today was ... and why ...

DATE .... HOW OLD IS BABY TODAY ...

Today is a tomorrow you worried about yesterday, and see ... everything's OK. —Anonymous

Prompt

Today I achieved ...

DATE .... HOW OLD IS BABY TODAY ...

A mother who has major surgery then comes home to care for a baby 24/7 is a super mum.

Prompt

I am most grateful for ...

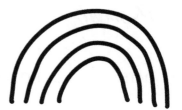

DATE .... HOW OLD IS BABY TODAY ...

Prompt

My baby fills my heart when ...

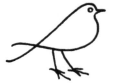

DATE .... HOW OLD IS BABY TODAY ...

The days are long but the years are short.—Gretchen Rubin

Prompt   I feel sad when ...

DATE .... HOW OLD IS BABY TODAY ...

Prompt

When I look at my scar, I feel ...

DATE .... HOW OLD IS BABY TODAY ...

Prompt

I would really appreciate help in ...

DATE .... HOW OLD IS BABY TODAY ...

Mindfulness is the key to peace and harmony ... one thing at a time.

Prompt

How will I fill my cup today ...

DATE .... HOW OLD IS BABY TODAY ...

To be a good parent, you need to take care of yourself so that you can have the physical and
emotional energy to take care of your family.' —Michelle Obama

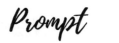

Prompt

The thing that hurts the most is ...

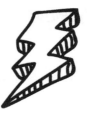

DATE .... HOW OLD IS BABY TODAY ...

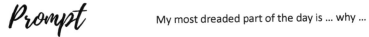

Prompt   My most dreaded part of the day is ... why ...

DATE .... HOW OLD IS BABY TODAY ...

Prompt

What I wish my partner understood is ...

DATE .... HOW OLD IS BABY TODAY ...

Prompt   I wish I had time for ...

DATE .... HOW OLD IS BABY TODAY ...

A mother's joy begins when new life is stirring inside ... when a tiny heartbeat is heard for the first time,
and a playful kick reminds her that she is never alone. —Author unknown

Prompt

I need to list my tasks I need help with. What is number 1 ...

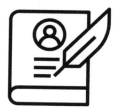

DATE .... HOW OLD IS BABY TODAY ...

Prompt

What am I most afraid of ...

DATE .... HOW OLD IS BABY TODAY ...

Prompt

What nourishment does my body need most now ...

DATE .... HOW OLD IS BABY TODAY ...

A baby will make love stronger, days shorter, nights longer, bankroll smaller, home happier, clothes shabbier, the past forgotten, and the future worth living for. —Anonymous

Prompt   If I could choose a song for my mantra today, what would it be ...

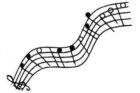

DATE .... HOW OLD IS BABY TODAY ...

Prompt   I laugh when I think of ...

DATE .... HOW OLD IS BABY TODAY ...

Prompt   What is my happiest memory about my baby's birth ...

Memories

DATE .... HOW OLD IS BABY TODAY ...

Mother's love is peace, it need not be acquired, it need not be deserved. —Erich Fromm

Prompt   If I had my time again, what would I like to change ...

DATE .... HOW OLD IS BABY TODAY ...

Mothers hold their children's hands for a while, but their hearts forever. —Author Unknown

Prompt

Today is going to be a good day because ...

DATE .... HOW OLD IS BABY TODAY ...

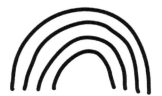

There is no way to be a perfect mother, but a million ways to be a good one. —Jill Churchill

Part Three
Daily Planners

✓ Your Daily Planner

Week One, Days 1—7 Use as your reminder

Week One Review	1	2	3	4	5	6	7
Bowels open? Bladder empty?							
Daily nap? Daily shower?							
Blood loss: Acceptable Heavy Offensive							
Breasts: Comfortable Engorged Painful							
Pain score monitoring 0—10							
Wound dressing removal as instructed? Clean and dry?							
• Daily nap							
• Set up help							
• Think Five layers							
• Scar inspection							
• Splint wound							
• Start journaling							
• Wear loose fitting clothes							
• Ease into postpartum							

Medications (Pain relief, vitamin D for breastfeeding mothers, etc.)	1	2	3	4	5	6	7

Food, snacks, and fluids	1	2	3	4	5	6	7
Breakfast and fluids							
Lunch and fluids							
Dinner and fluids							

Top Tips:

* Mindfully and leisurely take time to cuddle your baby, nurture and bond without rushing.
* Don't expect to bounce back quickly—you've had major surgery and need to recover slowly.
* Take all prescribed medication & supplements.
* Wear TED anti-clotting stockings.
* Check daily planners for your recovery checklist.
* Pour warm water between your legs after you pee and poo.
* Moisturise/massage IV sites.
* Keep medical contact numbers handy, just in case!

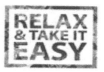

✓ Your Daily Planner

Week Two, Days 8—14 Use as your reminder

Week Two Review	8	9	10	11	12	13	14
Bowels settled? Bladder settled?							
Keep up daily nap and shower?							
Blood loss: Acceptable Heavy—observe Offensive—seek medical advice							
Breasts: Comfortable Engorged Painful							
Pain score monitoring 0—10							
Wound: keep clean and dry. Has it been reviewed by medics?							
• Continue help/support							
• Think Five layers							
• Scar inspection							
• Splint wound							
• Keep journaling							
• Wear loose fitting clothes							
• Ease into postpartum							

Medications (Pain relief, vitamin D for breastfeeding mothers, etc.)	8	9	10	11	12	13	14

Food, snacks, and fluids	8	9	10	11	12	13	14
Breakfast and fluids							
Lunch and fluids							
Dinner and fluids							

Top Tips:

- Mindfully and leisurely take time to cuddle your baby, nurture and bond without rushing.
- Don't expect to bounce back quickly—you've had major surgery and need to recover slowly.
- Take all prescribed medication & supplements.
- Mobilise a little more in the house and garden.
- Check daily planners for your recovery checklist.
- Baby weight?
- Baby had their heel prick screening?
- Keep medical contact numbers handy, just in case!

✓ Your Daily Planner

Week Three, Days 15–21 Use as your reminder

Week Three Review	15	16	17	18	19	20	21
Bowels normal? Bladder normal?							
Keep up daily nap and shower?							
Blood loss: Acceptable?							
Breasts: Comfortable?							
Pain score monitoring 0–10							
Wound clean and dry? View with a mirror. Gently massage. Any bruising?							
• Continue help/support							
• Think Five layers							
• Keep journaling							
• Wear loose fitting clothes							
• Ease into postpartum							

Medications (Pain relief, vitamin D for breastfeeding mothers, etc.)	15	16	17	18	19	20	21

Food, snacks, and fluids	15	16	17	18	19	20	21
Breakfast and fluids							
Lunch and fluids							
Dinner and fluids							

Top Tips:

* Mindfully and leisurely take time to cuddle your baby, nurture and bond without rushing.
* Don't expect to bounce back quickly—you've had major surgery and need to recover slowly.
* Take all prescribed medication & supplements.
* Enjoy a trip out with baby in a stroller.
* Check daily planners for your recovery checklist.
* Reflect on your recovery weeks 1–2.
* Pay attention to your emotional wellbeing.
* Keep medical contact numbers handy, just in case!

✓ Your Daily Planner

Week Four, Days 22–28 Use as your reminder

Week Four Review	22	23	24	25	26	27	28
Bowels normal? Bladder normal?							
Keep up daily nap and shower?							
Blood loss: Acceptable? Any concerns, seek medical support.							
Breasts: Comfortable?							
Pain score monitoring 0–10							
Wound clean and dry? View with a mirror. Gently massage. Any bruising? Any concerns, seek medical attention.							
• Continue help/support							
• Think Five layers							
• 5–6 weeks healing.							
• Keep journaling							
• Wear loose fitting clothes							
• Ease into postpartum							

Medications (Pain relief, vitamin D for breastfeeding mothers, etc.)	22	23	24	25	26	27	28

Food, snacks, and fluids	22	23	24	25	26	27	28
Breakfast and fluids							
Lunch and fluids							
Dinner and fluids							

Top Tips:

* Mindfully and leisurely take time to cuddle your baby, nurture and bond without rushing.
* Don't expect to bounce back quickly—you've had major surgery and need to recover slowly.
* Enjoy a trip out with baby in a stroller.
* Take all prescribed medication & supplements.
* Check daily planners for your recovery checklist.
* Reflect on your recovery weeks 1–3.
* Pay attention to your emotional wellbeing.
* Accept your new body image.
* Have you been debriefed on your birth?
* Book a salon pamper appointment.
* Keep your willing helpers a few weeks more.
* If not breastfeeding, observe monthly period.
* Keep medical contact numbers handy, just in case!
* Consider contraceptive choices.

✓ Your Daily Planner

Week Five, Days 29—35 Use as your reminder

Week Five Review	29	30	31	32	33	34	35
Bowels normal? Bladder normal?							
Keep up daily nap and shower?							
Blood loss: Acceptable? Any concerns, seek medical support.							
Breasts: Comfortable?							
Pain score monitoring 0—10							
Wound clean and dry? View with a mirror. Gently massage. Any bruising? Any concerns, seek medical attention.							
• Continue help/support							
• Think Five layers							
• 5–6 weeks healing.							
• Keep journaling							
• Wear loose fitting clothes							
• Ease into postpartum							

Medications (Pain relief, vitamin D for breastfeeding mothers, etc.)	29	30	31	32	33	34	35

Food, snacks, and fluids	29	30	31	32	33	34	35
Breakfast and fluids							
Lunch and fluids							
Dinner and fluids							

Top Tips:

* Mindfully and leisurely take time to cuddle your baby, nurture and bond without rushing.
* Don't expect to bounce back quickly—you've had major surgery and need to recover slowly.
* Enjoy a trip out with baby in a stroller.
* Take all prescribed medication & supplements.
* Check daily planners for your recovery checklist.
* Reflect on your recovery weeks 1–4.
* Pay attention to your emotional wellbeing.
* Accept your new body image.
* Have you been debriefed on your birth?
* Escape to the salon!
* Keep your willing helpers a few weeks more.
* If not breastfeeding, observe monthly period.
* Keep medical contact numbers handy, just in case!
* Consider contraceptive choices/date night.

✓ Your Daily Planner

Week Six, Days 36—42 Use as your reminder

Week Six Review	36	37	38	39	40	41	42
Bowels normal? Bladder normal?							
Keep up daily nap and shower? Enjoy the new you!							
Blood loss: any concerns, seek medical support.							
Breasts: do breast checks.							
Scar healing well?							
Consider your next cervical screening. Book your smear/postnatal review.							
• Prepare thank-you notes for your willing helpers.							
• Think Five layers							
• 6 weeks healing—still no heavy lifting.							
• Reflect on your journaling							
• Embrace your new body image.							
• Start light household duties.							

Medications (Pain relief, vitamin D for breastfeeding mothers, etc.)	36	37	38	39	40	41	42

Food, snacks, and fluids	36	37	38	39	40	41	42
Breakfast and fluids							
Lunch and fluids							
Dinner and fluids							

Top Tips:

* Mindfully and leisurely take time to cuddle your baby, nurture and bond without rushing.
* Don't expect to bounce back quickly—you've had major surgery and need to recover slowly.
* Enjoy a trip out with baby in a stroller.
* Take all prescribed medication & supplements.
* Check daily planners for your recovery checklist.
* Reflect on your recovery weeks 1–5.
* Pay attention to your emotional wellbeing.
* Is baby registered?
* Arrange baby immunisations.
* Think about driving again.
* Keep your willing helpers a few weeks more.
* If not breastfeeding, observe monthly period.
* Keep medical contact numbers at hand, just in case!
* Consider contraceptive choices/date night.

Appendices

Appendix 1
Caesarcare Scar Tracker

DAILY SCAR TRACKER

Normal pattern of healing

* Clean dry, pink/red suture line
* No swelling, pain, minor fluid loss
* No fever, no odour, no swelling
* Pain score reducing
* Possibly some wound itching

Abnormal Signs and Symptoms

* Fever
* Wound is hot, red, and painful
* Wound is oozing copious fluids
* An offensive odour from wound

If you experience abnormal signs and symptoms: SEEK MEDICAL REVIEW

Use this Scar Tracker to view, record, and decide on what to do if you suspect your wound is not healing as well as you would expect. Use the indicators above to record in the day tracker your findings. Seek medical opinion if you suspect a wound infection or breakdown. It is easier to use a hand-held mirror to observe your wound. Some wound dressings are time specific in their removal.

30 Day Scar Tracker
Describe your scar and decide if you need a review

1	2	3
4	5	6
7	8	9
10	11	12
13	14	15
16	17	18
19	20	21
22	23	24
25	26	27
28	29	30

Appendix 2
Scar Care Tips

Solicit support to help with cooking nutritious meals, washing, childminding, shopping, cleaning, carpooling, driving, naps, and visiting hours. It's a good idea to make a note on the door 'mother and baby sleeping, thank you for visiting'.

Control pain and take prescribed meds regularly to avoid peaks in pain score. Use ice to reduce inflammation. Control constipation with dietary fibre and plenty of fluids. Splint the wound with a cushion or rolled towel to control pressure on stitches during sudden movements such as coughing and sneezing.

Avoid tension on the stitches from a full bladder causing pressure on the internal stitches. Avoid coughing and too much laughter! Avoid lifting anything heavier than the baby, bending, hanging washing, and emptying baby bathwater. A long pick-up gadget is handy here. Contamination from dirty hands, soaked dressing, clean as required with mild soap and dress with a dry dressing. Don't dry with a hairdryer to avoid infection and damage to the tissues. Avoid friction from underwear or outer clothes by placing a pad in between.

Review and report any signs of infection, redness, swelling, odour, or temperature in your wound. Review your daily intake of nutrition and fluid, and drink at least 1.5 litres of water daily. Vitamin C is good for tissue repair. Use a daily checklist to track scar progress, medication, and food intake. Reflect on your emotional health and mindset be sure to debrief with a postnatal therapist if there is anything troubling you and causing you to feel stuck. Remember to support your stitches with a cushion or rolled towel during sudden movements.

Appendix 3
Gift ideas

GIFT IDEAS FOR MUMS AFTER CAESAREAN BIRTH

Here's a little list of some gift ideas for a post-C-Section mum.
The things that she'd REALLY love, but she's too polite to ever ask for!

1 Meal service.

2 Laundry service.

3 Time for a nap.

4 Underwear that doesn't mess up her scar.

5 Little luxuries.

6 Boring yet practical gifts from the local pharmacy.

7 The gift of a cleaner/house angel.

8 An I.O.U for an amazing night out. One day.

9 No visitors without calling first.

10 If in doubt: hand cream. Or face cream. Or fancy shampoo.
... and, of course, don't forget this C-section recovery book!

Resources

In both the UK and Australia, there are many resources available relating to childbirth and early parenting, and the list is forever growing and changing depending on funding and resources that are available. Few support groups are specifically for C-section recovery, mainly found on social media that can be helpful for families living in rural or isolated settings. Services fluctuate as a natural matter of course, as do contact details, websites and name changes, making it impossible to ensure lists of organisations are up to date and relevant in hard copy. An electronic copy is always the best means of getting current information and contact details.

The aim of the following is to signpost the let you know the primary services that are available for childbirth and early parenting support. Phone numbers and website addresses were correct at the time of publication (2022).

We would also suggest you use the following resources to find out what's around in your area and how to contact the specified service you need:

Australia
Your child and family health centre
This service is also called Maternal and Child Health and Child and Adolescent and Family Health, depending on the state you live in.

Telehealth nationwide AU1800 022 222
The child and family health centre is the first step for any concerns relating to your baby's development, health, or behaviour.

Your family doctors

The maternity hospital

Your nearest community health centre

Free services from nurses, psychologists, social workers, counsellors, speech pathologists, and psychiatrists work from community health centres, but there can be long waiting lists. Information about private services is available from community health centres, your family doctor, and child and family health nurses.

Your nearest children's or local hospital

A variety of free services available via the public hospital system, including paediatric dietitians, occupational therapists, speech pathologists, psychologists, physiotherapists, optometrists, audiologists, and more. Again, depending on the urgency and the service, there can be long waits. Some children's hospitals have twenty-four-hour helplines to answer questions about childhood illnesses.

Your local council

Postnatal Physiotherapy Information for Aboriginal Women

Your local library

Phone book for the capital city of your state

Mensline: 1300 789 978

www.panda.org.au PTSD

Dietitians Association of Australia (DAA)

If you need an accredited dietitian and don't know where to go, call 1800 812 942 to obtain names and contact details. Make sure you let them know it's for paediatric advice.

www.daa.asn.au

Domestic violence

Advice and resources vary from state to state. Look in the front of the White Pages for contact numbers in your state. Numbers include emergency help, advocacy services, and local community services.

A national confidential domestic violence helpline is available on 1800 200 526.

Parent education

The availability and range of parent education varies widely across Australia. It is often available via child and family health centres, community health centres, extended day care centres, schools, children's hospitals, churches, residential family and baby centres, associations such as the ABA, AMBA, Playgroup Association of Australia, and local councils.

Finding out what is available is usually a challenge. Local newspapers often advertise parent education courses/functions. Try a Google search if you are on the net. A useful resource is the website of the Children's Hospital at Westmead in Sydney.

United Kingdom
GP/ Health Visitor/ midwife

Community Health Services

Child Health Services 0–19 years of age

Breastfeeding Support Networks

Children's Centres

Birth Debrief services via your delivering hospital team

Patient Liaison Services, via your medical institution

NHS .Net online health services <https://www.nhs.uk/health-at-home/>

<https://www.nesta.org.uk/feature/everyday-social-innovations/the-national-childbirth-trust/>

National Health Services online services

National Institute of Clinical Excellence

Royal College of Midwifery

Facebook chat pages

Mumsnet <https://www.mumsnet.com/>

Tommy's <https://www.tommys.org/>

Breastfeeding world health organisation <https://www.who.int/health-topics/breastfeeding>

Maternal mental health services <https://www.england.nhs.uk/mental-health/perinatal/>

Lullaby trust <https://www.lullabytrust.org.uk/>

Dad Info <https://www.dad.info/>

Domestic abuse <https://www.nationaldahelpline.org.uk/>

Children's centres <https://www.gov.uk/find-sure-start-childrens-centre>

NHS111 <https://www.nhs.uk/using-the-nhs/nhs-services/urgent-and-emergency-care/nhs-111/>

Social services UK <https://www.nhs.uk/conditions/social-care-and-support-guide/>

SANDS Stillbirth and Neonatal Death Charity <https://www.sands.org.uk/&p=1&pos=1>

Miscarriage charity <https://www.miscarriageassociation.org.uk/about-us/the-charity/>

Caesarean section support <https://www.nhs.uk/conditions/caesarean-section/recovery/>

DVLA driving after birth <https://www.gov.uk/guidance/miscellaneous-conditions-assessing-fitness-to-drive>

Global
<www.ican-online.org>
<www.specialscars.org>

Glossary

adhesions—When a woman's body recovers after the surgical procedure of C-section, it can form a set of scar tissue known as adhesions.

anaemia—a deficiency in the number or quality of red blood cells in your body. Red blood cells carry oxygen around your body using a particular protein called haemoglobin. Anaemia means that either the level of red blood cells or the level of haemoglobin is lower than normal.

anaesthetic—a drug that gives total or partial loss of sensation of a part or the whole of the body.

anaesthetist—a doctor who specialises in giving anaesthetic.

analgesics—a class of drugs used to relieve analgesia (pain). They work by blocking pain signals to the brain or interfering with the brain's interpretation of those signals. Analgesics are broadly categorised as being either non-opioid (non-narcotic) or opioid (narcotic) pain relievers.

antenatal—a term that means 'before birth' (alternative terms are 'prenatal' and 'antepartum').

antepartum haemorrhage—bleeding from the vagina during pregnancy.

APGAR score—a test given one minute after a baby is born, then again five minutes later, that assesses a baby's *appearance* (skin colour), *pulse*, *grimace* (reflex), *activity* (muscle tone), and *respiration*. A perfect APGAR score is 10; typical APGAR scores are seven, eight, or nine. A score lower than seven means that the baby might need help breathing.

baby blues—mild depression that follows childbirth; usually the result of hormonal swings.

birth plan—a written document describing a woman's preferences for her care during labour and birth.

blood transfusion—a procedure where a woman is given blood.

breech—when the baby is positioned inside the uterus with its bottom or feet down, instead of its head.

caesarean section—a surgical procedure in which a baby is delivered through a cut in the abdomen and uterus (also called a 'C-section').

colostrum—(also known as 'beestings' or 'first milk') is a form of milk produced by the mammary glands in late pregnancy and the few days after giving birth.

continuity of care—care from a known midwife is often referred to as midwifery continuity of care. Women who have the same midwife caring for them throughout pregnancy, labour, birth, and post-birth have the opportunity to build a trusting relationship which increases their confidence.

epidural—a type of anaesthetic commonly used in labour where drugs are used to numb the lower half of the body.

fertility—being able to conceive and carry a baby through to the end of the pregnancy.

first trimester—the first 14 weeks of pregnancy.

fontanelles—the six soft spots on a baby's head that allow its skull to compress during birth so it can pass through the birth canal. The fontanels completely fuse by the time the child is two years old.

full term—when a pregnancy is a normal duration (37–42 weeks gestation).

gestation—the length of time (in days or weeks) that a baby is in the uterus.

gestational diabetes—a condition that develops during pregnancy when the woman's blood sugar levels become too high because of inadequate levels of insulin. The condition is treatable and usually disappears after pregnancy.

gynaecologist—a doctor who has undertaken specialist training in women's health.

haemorrhage—excessive bleeding.

in utero—a term that means 'inside the uterus'.

incontinence—an inability to control your bladder or bowel movements.

induced—when a healthcare professional tries to artificially 'start' a woman's labour.

jaundice—a condition where a person's skin and the whites of their eyes take on a yellowish tinge. It is caused by an excess of a chemical called bilirubin in the blood and in newborns often resolves itself.

lactation consultant—a healthcare professional who is trained to provide information and support about breastfeeding.

low birthweight—when a baby weighs less than 2,500 grams at birth.

maternal and child health nurse—a trained nurse who specialises in the health and development of children from birth to school age.

meconium—a tar-like substance passed by a baby as their first poo. Passing meconium before birth may be a sign of foetal distress.

midwife—a person who has been specially trained to care for women during pregnancy, labour, birth, and the post-birth period.

model of care—the way maternity care is organised.

multiple pregnancy—when a woman is carrying more than one baby.

natural birth—birth without any interventions for example a vaginal birth rather than a caesarean section.

neonatal period—the time from a baby's birth to four weeks of age.

neonatal intensive care unit (NICU)—a unit in the hospital for babies who need a high level of special medical care.

neonate—a newborn baby, up to four weeks of age.

newborn—a baby between birth and four weeks old.

nursery—a room in a hospital where babies can stay during the day or overnight.

obstetrician—a doctor who has undertaken specialist training in pregnancy and childbirth.

paediatrician—a doctor who has undertaken specialist training in treating children.

pelvic floor exercises—exercises a woman can do to strengthen the muscles in and around her vagina.

Glossary

placenta—the organ that connects to the wall of the uterus, that nourishes the baby through the umbilical cord.

placenta accreta—occurs when the placenta grows too deeply into the uterine wall.

placenta increta—a condition where the placenta attaches more firmly to the uterus and becomes embedded in the organ's muscle wall. Placenta accreta is a condition where placenta attaches itself and grows through the uterus and potentially to the nearby organs (such as the bladder).

postnatal—a term meaning 'after birth' (alternative terms are 'post-birth' and 'postpartum').

postpartum depression—a condition that affects some mothers in the days, weeks, or months after giving birth.

postpartum haemorrhage—when a woman loses more than 500 ml of blood after birth.

pre-eclampsia—a pregnancy complication characterised by high blood pressure and signs of damage to another organ system, most often the liver and kidneys. Pre-eclampsia usually begins after twenty weeks of pregnancy in women whose blood pressure had been normal.

premature—when a baby is born before 37 weeks gestation.

prenatal—a term meaning 'before birth' (alternative terms are 'antenatal' and 'antepartum').

second-degree tear—a tear of the perineum involving both skin and muscles, but not the anus. Second-degree tears often require stitches.

second-stage labour—the time from the complete dilation of the cervix (ten centimetres) to the birth.

second trimester—the time from 14 weeks to 26 weeks of pregnancy.

sepsis—a potentially life-threatening condition caused by the body's response to an infection. The body normally releases chemicals into the bloodstream to fight infection. Sepsis occurs when the body's response to these chemicals is out of balance, triggering changes that can damage multiple organ systems.

special care nursery (SCN)—a unit in a hospital for babies who need special medical care.

spontaneous labour—when labour starts by itself (without medical help).

stillbirth—the death of a baby after 20 weeks gestation but before birth.

stretch marks—discoloured stripey patterns that can appear on the abdomen, breasts, buttocks, or legs during pregnancy because of skin stretching. They usually fade slowly after birth.

TENS machine—a 'transcutaneous electrical nerve stimulation' machine used for pain management during labour.

theatre—an operating room in a hospital or other health facility.

third- or fourth-degree tear—a severe tear of the perineum involving the skin, muscles, and anus. Stitches are used to repair these tears.

third trimester—the time from 26 weeks of pregnancy onwards.

TOLAC—Trial of Labour after Caesarean birth.

trimester—a time span of three months during pregnancy, each marked by different phases of foetal development.

uterus—a woman's womb.

vacuum cap or ventouse—a suction cap that is sometimes used during birth to help to pull the baby out of the birth canal.

VBAC (vaginal birth after caesarean)—when a woman has a vaginal birth after having had one or more previous caesarean sections.

walking epidural—an epidural that may still enable the woman to walk.

waters—the amniotic fluid that surrounds an unborn baby inside the uterus (see 'amniotic fluid').

woman-centred care—woman-centred care focuses on the woman's unique needs, expectations, and aspirations; recognises her right to self-determination in terms of choice, control and continuity of care; and addresses her social, emotional, physical, psychological, spiritual, and cultural needs and expectations (NMBA 2006).

wound dehiscence—a partial or total separation of previously approximated **wound** edges, due to a failure of proper **wound** healing.

Index